An End to Upside Down Medicine

Also by Mark Gober

AN END TO UPSIDE DOWN THINKING

Dispelling the Myth That the Brain Produces Consciousness, and the Implications for Everyday Life

AN END TO UPSIDE DOWN LIVING

Reorienting Our Consciousness to Live Better and Save the Human Species

AN END TO UPSIDE DOWN LIBERTY

Turning Traditional Political Thinking on Its Head to Break Free from Enslavement

AN END TO UPSIDE DOWN CONTACT

UFOs, Aliens, and Spirits—and Why Their Ongoing Interaction with Human Civilization Matters

AN END TO THE UPSIDE DOWN RESET

The Leftist Vision for Society Under the "Great Reset"—and How It Can Fool Caring People into Supporting Harmful Causes

Note from the author: Throughout, I have slightly edited some quoted material for spelling, punctuation, and clarity. "Emphasis added" is noted when I have added bold or italics in a particular paragraph. If this is not noted, it means that any bold or italics were in the original. Also, please note that I am not a doctor. The concepts discussed in this book are for informational and educational purposes only. They do not constitute medical advice. Before embarking on new explorations for one's own health, please consult a medical practitioner.

An End to Upside Down Medicine

Contagion, Viruses, and Vaccines—and Why Consciousness Is Needed for a New Paradigm of Health

Mark Gober

Waterside Productions
Cardiff-by-the-Sea, California

The graph showing pesticide use over time versus polio incidence in chapter 4 has been re-created with the permission of Jim West at harvoa.org and one of the original publishers of the data, the Weston A. Price Foundation, at https://www.westonaprice.org/health-topics/environmental-toxins/pesticides-and-polio-a-critique-of-scientific-literature/#gsc.tab=0. The graphs showing trends of deaths caused by various diseases relative to the introduction of a vaccine in chapter 5 have been re-created with the permission of Roman Bystrianyk, the co-author of *Dissolving Illusions* (2013), and the charts are also publicly available at: https://dissolvingillusions.com/graphs-images/#Charts. The United States childhood-vaccination schedule in chapter 5 has been re-created with permission from Skyhorse Publishing, the publisher of *Vax-Unvax: Let the Science Speak* (2023). The longer-than-normal quotation from Dr. Samantha Bailey's 2021 video explaining a 2003 SARS study has been printed with her permission. The video version is available at her website: https://drsambailey.com/; and her Odysee channel, https://odysee.com/@drsambailey:c/what-happened-to-sars-1:8.

First Printing, 2023
Printed in the United States of America

ISBN-13: 978-1-960583-86-4 print edition
ISBN-13: 978-1-960583-87-1 ebook edition
ISBN-13: 979-8-212980-73-9 audiobook edition

Waterside Productions
2055 Oxford Avenue
Cardiff-by-the-Sea, CA 92007
www.waterside.com

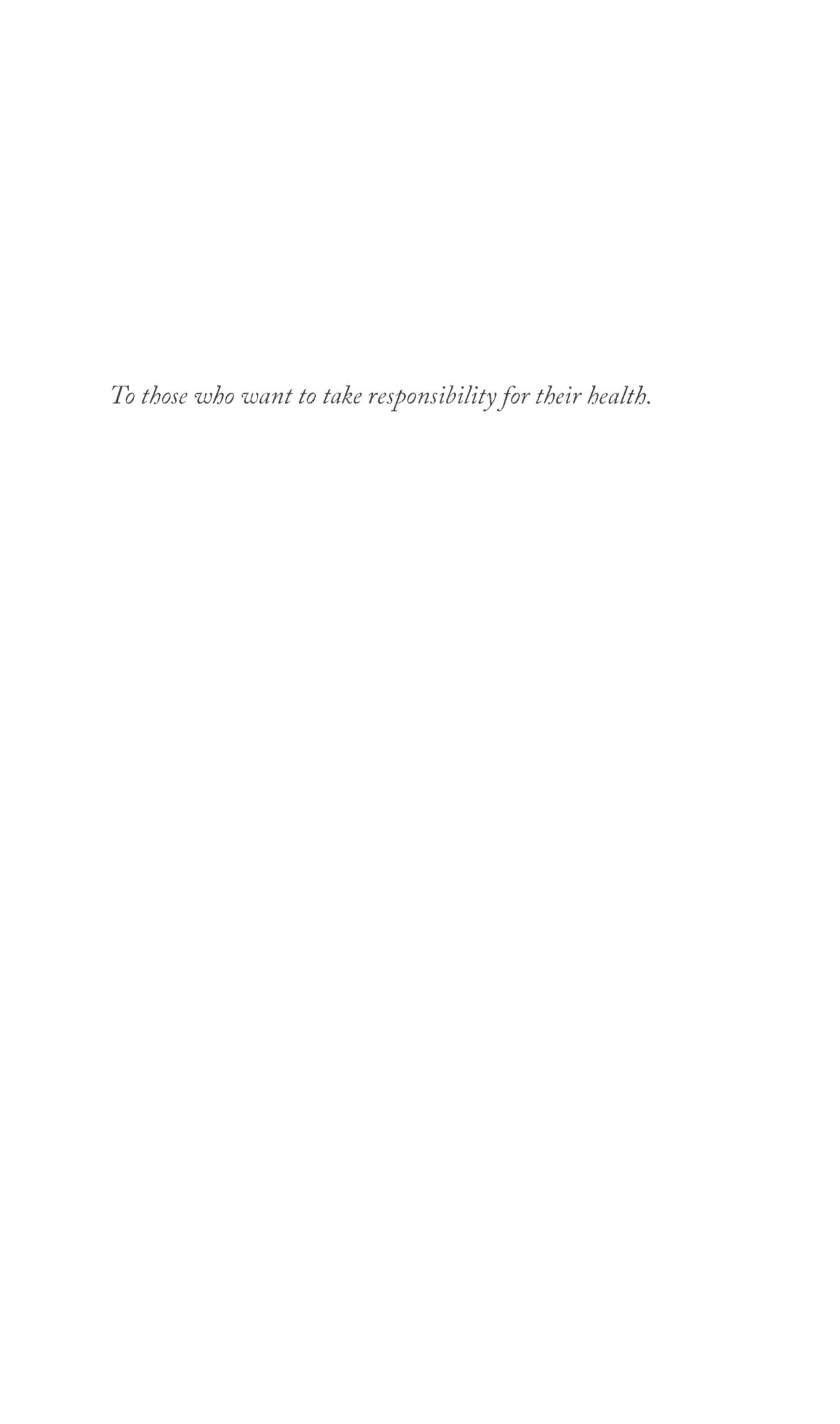

To those who want to take responsibility for their health.

"Some things are believed because they are demonstrably true. But many other things are believed simply because they have been asserted repeatedly—and repetition has been accepted as a substitute for evidence."

—Economist Thomas Sowell[1]

CONTENTS

PART II
WHY IS CONSCIOUSNESS RELEVANT TO MEDICINE?

INTRODUCTION

ALLOPATHIC MEDICINE AND THE HURDLES TO OVERCOMING IT

According to the Centers for Disease Control and Prevention (CDC), 60 percent of American adults have at least one chronic disease, and 40 percent have two or more chronic diseases.[1] The CDC also notes that heart disease is the leading cause of death in the United States.[2] Yet, in the early 20th century, death from heart disease was rare.[3] Cancer is the second-leading cause of death. This comes more than fifty years after President Richard Nixon's 1971 declaration of a "War on Cancer,"[4] in which scientists were looking for a virus that caused the disease.[5] Countless billions of dollars have been invested, and yet cancer is not well understood. The third-leading cause of death is "unintentional injury."[6] Although the CDC's report doesn't elaborate on this category beyond a reference to drug overdoses, many researchers have similarly suggested that "iatrogenesis" is the third-leading cause of death: instances in which *the medical profession* caused death.[7] As stated by Rafia Farooq Peer and Nadeem Shabir in a 2018 article published in the *Journal of Family Medicine and Primary Care*, "Iatrogenic ailments are those where doctors, drugs, diagnostics, hospitals, and other medical institutions act as 'pathogens' or 'sickening agents.'"[8] In his book *Death by Medicine* (2011), Gary Null, PhD, notes that "as little as 5% and no more than 20% of iatrogenic events are ever reported."[9] So the number of deaths caused by the medical profession is likely quite significant.

Modern medicine isn't working.

The primary aim of this book is to shine light on the core flaws of the mainstream Western approach to health—known as *allopathic medicine*—and instead point toward a new and improved paradigm. The current model is actively perpetuated by the pharmaceutical industry, doctors, the media, politicians, and academia, while many everyday citizens go along with it without asking questions. This topic is of paramount importance, because without being healthy, we can't live our best lives. And as many of us have experienced during the COVID-19 era, a declared public health emergency can be weaponized to enact tyrannical measures on a global scale. If we want to be free, both individually and collectively, we need to get medicine right.

Before exploring specific—and radical—critiques of allopathy, in this introductory chapter I will set the stage by examining the underlying dynamics that enable the status quo.

What Is Allopathic Medicine?

The allopathic approach can be summarized by its two core and interrelated tenets: (1) reductionism, and (2) a focus on symptoms rather than solving the root causes of disease.

Allopathic medicine is reductionistic in that it often reduces a set of symptoms to a single, tangible cause that can be cured by a single pharmaceutical treatment, rather than considering a mosaic of causes and natural treatment modalities. **It can be summarized as "one disease, one cause, one miracle pill."**[10] The approach is not holistic. [emphasis added]

The allopathic model also ignores—or even ridicules—the possibility of the "soul" or the existence of "spiritual dimensions" inherent in our reality, despite a substantial body of scientific evidence to the contrary (as will be discussed later). That is, modern medicine reduces the nature of reality—and biology—to physical particles. This flawed philosophy is known as *physicalism* or *scientific materialism*. It's difficult to get medicine right without first properly considering what a human being is.

Moreover, all too often, allopathic treatment simply entails finding a physical enemy to eradicate—such as bacteria and viruses. Under this ethos, health problems are best managed with drugs, prevented with vaccines, or removed by surgery.

The reductionistic approach also implicitly views humans as biological robots who are destined to have certain ailments because of their genetics, and there's nothing they can do about it. The name for such a belief is *genetic determinism*.[11] This often-unstated perspective neglects the emerging field of epigenetics, which suggests that genetic activity isn't fixed; rather, it is impacted by factors in one's environment. *The Biology of Belief* (2005), the groundbreaking book by Bruce Lipton, PhD, popularized this concept. More broadly, our understanding of genetics and heredity is in its infancy, and there is likely much that we don't know.

In addition to being reductionistic, allopathic medicine often fails to arrive at the root causes of disease and instead tries to eradicate symptoms. This approach can be effective for emergency situations—where the allopathic approach is certainly valuable, and, at times, lifesaving. **But under allopathy, this "emergency" approach is applied broadly; it is the rule rather than the exception.** As stated by Suzanne Humphries, MD: "[I've] witnessed the miracles of giving someone a drug when [patients] need it.... The problem is that when people have minor health issues, this kind of medicine is used automatically as the first line of defense. And none of these drugs from the pharmaceutical industry bring people to higher states of natural health. Whereas there are many [other supplements] and nutritional advice [that can allow people] to avoid these drugs."[12]

The majority of modern medicine thus serves as a "Band-Aid," solving a problem in the short term but leaving open the potential for persistent, long-term ailments. By suppressing symptoms, the drugs might even be hindering the body's natural healing process, and it's difficult to know how damaging that is. Thus, many patients end up taking pharmaceutical drugs indefinitely, and most of the time they don't even know what the chemicals are inside the pills. And since drugs typically have side effects—some of which are known and others that are perhaps not yet recognized—new symptoms can emerge that warrant additional pharmaceutical drugs. The cycle can be ongoing until the patient dies.

Pharmaceutical Dominance

The pharmaceutical industry—and the doctors who sell its products—perpetuate the flawed allopathic model. This inertia explains why it's been so difficult for nonallopathic modes of treatment to gain traction.

Consider this issue from a strictly financial perspective: Long-term pharmaceutical prescriptions are great for drug companies' bottom lines. Curing people quickly makes far less money than having a customer for the duration of his or her lifetime. It's just math.

Moreover, the allopathic approach leads to dependence on the pharmaceutical industry. That's good for pharmaceutical profitability but not so good for individual freedom. **Thus, everyday people are discouraged from taking responsibility for their own health outside of the "system."**

We saw this very clearly during the COVID-19 era that began in 2020. The messaging from health authorities was not to focus on nutrition, sleep, exercise, natural sunlight, relationships, a healthy mental state, or alternative treatment modalities. Rather, the public was told to be afraid, avoid people, wear masks that restrict airflow and contain harmful chemicals,[13] stay indoors, and wait for pharmaceutical pills and vaccines to save the day. The godlike saviors were the "experts" and the pharmaceutical companies; essentially, they became priests of a religion. In fact, nonpharmaceutical solutions were actively condemned, or their advocates were branded as heretical "conspiracy theorists."

Beyond what we saw around COVID-19, the cultural milieu against nonallopathic medicine is pervasive. Doctors who don't follow the traditional script are often reflexively called "quacks." This messaging is amplified by the pharmaceutical-influenced media, in part because they are such big advertisers.[14] (Note: Regarding television specifically, this dynamic only applies in the United States and New Zealand. As of 2023, pharmaceutical companies are still allowed to advertise their prescription drugs directly to consumers in those two countries, whereas elsewhere this is not allowed.[15])

In 1910, the general attitude toward medicine changed in the United States and Canada with the release of a lengthy report by Abraham Flexner. It was issued by the Carnegie Foundation and supported by the Rockefeller Foundation.[16] The Flexner Report advocated for an overhaul of the medical system and dismissed "the homeopathists [*sic*], the eclectics, the physiomedicals, and the osteopaths"[17] in favor of a widespread allopathic model. As noted in a 2011 paper titled "The Flexner Report—100 Years Later"—written by Thomas Duffy, MD, and published in the *Yale Journal of Biology and Medicine,* the Flexner report "transformed the nature and process of medical education in America with a resulting elimination of proprietary schools and the establishment of the biomedical model as the gold standard of medical training." Two years later, Flexner published a similar critique of the medical systems in France, Britain, and Germany.[18]

Furthermore, allopathic education has been heavily influenced by the pharmaceutical industry, which pours millions of dollars into medical schools.[19] Naturally, this dynamic can shape doctors' opinions as well as the types of drugs they'll prescribe. Emergency physician Joel Lexchin, MD, MS, notes that "[drug companies] make contact early on with medical students when these students are at an impressionable time in terms of their professional life.... [These] companies want to establish a positive relationship with these medical students that can then go forward."[20] Dr. Lexchin also notes that by giving money to medical schools, pharmaceutical companies build relationships with the faculty, which in effect enables them to mold students into the types of doctors that the industry wants them to be.[21]

Dr. Humphries elaborates on this point: **"[Later in my career,] I realized something that I didn't realize before I went to medical school, which is that what I had really become was a highly trained technician for the pharmaceutical industry.** And this was saddening to me because my original intention was to go and be able to heal people and cure their diseases and bring them to higher levels of health. And I didn't learn to do that in medical school."[22] [emphasis added]

The pharmaceutical industry is naturally incentivized to steer not just medical education, but also research, toward allopathic solutions. That means there is less funding for "alternative" medical treatments. And that means fewer studies. Therefore, the experts can claim that "there's not enough evidence that these other treatments are effective; the data just isn't there." Would they be able to make this claim if holistic medicine had the same level of funding—and amount of formal research—that the allopathic model has?

Along these lines, the pharmaceutical industry is motivated to prioritize the funding of studies that affirm the safety and efficacy of their products. And having their tentacles in the regulatory process itself is critical. As reported in a 2021 article published by the University of Connecticut, almost half of the US government's Food and Drug Administration (FDA) budget comes from pharmaceutical companies themselves[23]—the very companies that the regulatory agency is supposed to be regulating. Making matters worse, as of 2019, nine out of the previous ten FDA commissioners joined pharmaceutical companies after leaving the FDA.[24] The system is incestuous.

Furthermore, the pharmaceutical industry's influence on politicians amplifies the problem. More than two-thirds of Congress took money from the pharmaceutical industry in 2020.[25] As aptly stated by journalist PJ O'Rourke, **"When buying and selling are**

controlled by legislation, the first things to be bought and sold are legislators."[26] [emphasis added]

These troubling trends aren't favorable to citizens. For example, consider the fact that the FDA has a history of approving drugs that are later pulled from the market because of safety concerns. What follows is a list of nearly forty examples: Accutane, Baycol, Belviq/Belviq XR, Bextra, Cylert, Darvon & Darvocet, DBI, DES, Duract, Ergamisol, Hismanal, Lotronex, Meridia, Merital & Alival, Micturin, Mylotarg, Omniflox, Palladone, Permax, Pondimin, Posicor, Propulsid, PTZ & Metrazol, Quaalude, Raplon, Raptiva, Raxar, Redux, Rezulin, Selacryn, Seldane, Trasylol, Vioxx, Xigris, Zantac, Zelmid, and Zelnorm.[27] One might wonder if some drugs initially made it through the regulatory process because of pressure from their key funders: pharmaceutical companies and the government (which is influenced by the pharmaceutical industry).

So, when published clinical evidence talks about how safe and effective a certain drug is, it's only rational for the public to be skeptical. John Abramson, MD, of Harvard Medical School; and Barbara Starfield, MD, of Johns Hopkins, even suggested that we "give up the illusion that the primary purpose of modern medical research is to improve Americans' health most effectively and efficiently.... **The primary purpose of commercially funded clinical research is to maximize financial return on investment, not health."**[28] And as stated by Peter Duesberg, PhD, a professor of molecular and cell biology at the University of California, Berkeley: "They're all prostitutes—most of them, my colleagues, [and] to some degree myself. You have to be a prostitute to get money for your research. You're trained a little bit to be a prostitute. But some go all the way."[29] [emphasis added]

Drug companies haven't been able to get away with everything, however. In physician Peter Gøtzcshe's 2017 book, *Deadly Medicines and Organised Crime: How Big Pharma Has Corrupted Healthcare*, he includes a list of major settlements paid by pharmaceutical companies that total in the billions of dollars. He writes: "I did 10 Google searches in 2012 combining the names of the 10 largest drug companies with 'fraud.' There were between 0.5 and

27 million hits for each company."[30] (Note: This was done back when Google searches were less biased. Now, it has become harder and harder to find "alternative" medical information using Google because the top search results tend to direct users to articles that fit the prevailing allopathic narrative.[31])

Doctor Problems

Although the field of allopathic medicine is filled with unsavory dynamics, many doctors do have good intentions.[32] The problem is that good intentions don't always mean good results. Often doctors become "order followers" and don't question the authority of the system. They have to work incredibly hard in competitive schools just to obtain their degrees, and in some cases, that could understandably lead to big egos and a lack of intellectual humility. Rigid belief systems can result—especially when combined with a pharmaceutical-influenced medical-school experience.

Doctors also have to worry about malpractice, which naturally pushes them toward conformity. And if they want to be practical about their finances, they need to weigh the risks and benefits of challenging conventions. Dr. Mark Bailey, a New Zealand–based physician, comments on the conundrum with which doctors are confronted:

> They face the choice of: speak out, but then lose your license and your money....Sometimes people put doctors on a pedestal, but they're just like everyone else. They get into debt, they have mortgages, they have car payments, they have businesses with huge overheads. And for most of them, the thought of [even] losing a paycheck is pretty hard to bear. Which is why you'll see they mainly comply and go along with things without a whimper no matter how tyrannical things get. And we saw that in the last couple of years [during the COVID-19 era]. Most of them would rather just stay completely silent rather than...say, "I'm going to question this."[33]

Mark Bailey's wife, Dr. Samantha Bailey, further reflects on dynamics that instill conformity based on her personal experience in the medical system:

> The most esteemed and rewarded colleagues are often those that could recite medical dogma most accurately. It was literally the way to win awards and secure so-called top positions in academic and clinical medicine. We were not encouraged to question the prescribed textbooks or published papers in peer-reviewed journals.... In general, we were expected to regurgitate the claims which were said to represent the highest level of scientific evidence....
>
> The problem with the medical system is that it was co-opted so long ago that nobody in generations has seen what a health system would look like. As one of my good friends says..."It is not a health system. It is a sick system."...The practitioners in many parts of the medical system may be hard working and think they're helping. But sadly they have been duped into paying homage to false models and often harm, if not kill, people....They are indoctrinated not to question the medical establishment and think that the "science" is on their side. It is clear that the majority of them do not critically appraise the evidence in their own practices.... In their minds, the science is decided by...the government, the corporate sponsors of the medical journals, and Facebook community guidelines.[34]

Finally, on a more insidious note, Dr. Gøtzcshe observes that "the industry buys friends....There is a culture among doctors that allows acceptance of easy money, and companies may offer to transfer the money in ways that cannot be traced....The truth is that by far most doctors assist the [pharmaceutical companies] in marketing their products."[35]

Psychological Hurdles

In addition to headwinds posed by the medical establishment, the general public's psychology serves as a barrier to a new medical paradigm. More specifically, the way people think often anchors them toward the prevailing and engrained belief systems.

So, before embarking on a journey to poke holes in the allopathic model, it's first important to appropriately orient one's mindset. This exercise aims to reduce the cognitive dissonance—emotional discomfort—that might accompany forthcoming discussions in this book.

1. *Anomalies matter.* An anomaly is something that doesn't fit a worldview. It is an exception to the rule.[36] Encountering *even a single anomaly* is problematic because it implies that the "rule" is incorrect, and a new one is needed. For instance, in 1900, one of the leading authorities in science, Lord Kelvin, declared that physics had largely figured things out, but there were two pesky "clouds"—unsolved mysteries—that remained. Upon further study, those clouds emerged into what are now known as relativity theory and quantum mechanics. Two anomalies resulted in drastic changes in scientific thinking.[37]

2. *Correlation does not imply causation.* If someone observes firefighters at the scene of a fire, there are multiple possible explanations. Without having any background knowledge, one might assume that the firefighters *caused* the fire. Alternatively, one might believe that the fire has a mystical ability to manifest humans out of thin air, so the firefighters are a by-product of the fire itself.[38] Of course, these explanations miss the correct reason, which is that firefighters appeared on the scene *in response to* the fire. The point here is that when two things are related to one another, or if they appear at the same place and at the same time, the relationship between those things needs to be explored carefully. That is, the correlation of

those things doesn't automatically imply that one *caused* the other. All possibilities need to be considered in order to accurately explain the relationship.

This point is critical in the exercise of uncovering the causes of illness. For instance, if people get sick in the same place around the same time, one can't automatically conclude that a contagious virus or bacteria *caused* it. Maybe the sick people were exposed to a common environmental toxin; or consumed food or water that contained toxins; or were exposed to a similar form of radiation or a dangerous electromagnetic field; or were affected by a change in seasons, humidity, temperature, or barometric pressure; or they were under similar emotional distress; or they were exposed to some other factor, or factors, that could collectively contribute to illness. Critical thinking and open-mindedness are thus essential in the process of exploring causation.

3. *Presuppositions often go unacknowledged.* A presupposition is an assumption that underlies a belief system. If presuppositions aren't examined, people end up believing things without knowing *why* they believe those things—other than "someone told me this was true." Consider the six-feet-social-distancing requirement that dominated policy around the world during the COVID-19 era. In 2021, former FDA commissioner Scott Gottlieb revealed to CBS that the rule was "arbitrary."[39] Yet, how many people religiously followed the rule, trusting that it would save lives because people on television said so? The belief that "it must be true because an expert said it" is a logical fallacy known as "appeal to authority." Cultlike superstitions are the result.

4. *Science is an approach, not a religion.* These days, the term *science* has come to refer to "anything that a mainstream scientist or doctor says." Anthony Fauci, MD, a leading public medical figure in the United States, even declared in 2021 that attacks on him are "attacks on

science."[40] In reality, the scientific method is supposed to be an approach that welcomes endless challenges, whereas religious dogma is not allowed to be questioned. The institution of "science," ironically, has become its own religion.

5. *Consensus does not always mean "truth."* There is often a belief that if the majority of authority figures believe something, then it must be true—as if it's not possible that so many prominent people could be wrong. Author Michael Crichton explained why this is such a problematic approach:

   > I regard consensus science as an extremely pernicious development that ought to be stopped cold in its tracks. Historically, the claim of consensus has been the first refuge of scoundrels; it is a way to avoid debate by claiming that the matter is already settled. Whenever you hear the consensus of scientists agrees on something or other, reach for your wallet, because you're being had....Let's be clear: the work of science has nothing whatever to do with consensus. Consensus is the business of politics. Science, on the contrary, requires only one investigator who happens to be right, which means that he or she has results that are verifiable by reference to the real world. In science, consensus is irrelevant. What is relevant is reproducible results. The greatest scientists in history are great precisely because they broke with the consensus. There is no such thing as consensus science. If it's consensus, it isn't science. If it's science, it isn't consensus. Period.[41]

What's to Come in This Book

With this contextual backdrop, I will move into an examination of flawed allopathic assumptions. Although I will discuss potential alternatives, they are presented in a hypothetical manner, and they need to be studied further.

Said another way, the ideas I discuss in this book should not be taken as definitive proof of anything. But, taken together, the pieces of evidence suggest that the allopathic approach is misguided—not just a *little* bit misguided, but *severely* misguided. That means we need to be looking for new models if we want to achieve better health. Therefore, it's necessary to consider ideas that are far outside of conventional thinking. And given how unhealthy modern society is, such a radical exercise is warranted.

Thus, the examination of the medical system in this book aspires to "start from scratch"—as if we know nothing about medicine and are exploring health and disease for the very first time. That entails asking the question: "How is it that we know the things we think we know? And how certain are we of those things?"

Keeping that approach in mind, in part I of this book I explore why allopathic assumptions need to be challenged. The first exploration, in chapter 1, takes a fresh look at HIV/AIDS. This serves as a template for later discussions about other diseases. Viruses—and how they are identified and "isolated"—are explored in chapter 2. The discussion walks through potential flaws built into the field of virology itself. Chapter 3 then sets the stage for a reevaluation of *all* allegedly infectious diseases by examining the logic needed to establish a cause of disease. That framework provides a backdrop with which to examine a variety of conditions commonly believed to be infectious, including polio, SARS, Spanish flu, avian flu, smallpox, chicken pox, hepatitis, rabies, and the Black Death (chapter 4). In the process of reviewing these illnesses, many questions about vaccines arise, which leads to a deeper analysis of their safety in chapter 5.

In part II, I explore consciousness and why it's a necessary component of a comprehensive medical model. In chapter 6, I dive into the nature of reality—and the human body's place in it—which presents a fundamental challenge to allopathic beliefs. The resulting framework makes way for a discussion about consciousness, health, and disease in chapter 7. The topics covered are so far outside of traditional thinking that they make modern medicine seem highly primitive.

I conclude this book with a discussion of what's at stake for all of us, in terms of our individual and collective freedom. The implications are immense.

PART I
WHY SHOULD ALLOPATHIC ASSUMPTIONS BE QUESTIONED?

CHAPTER 1
HIV/AIDS

Allopathic medicine's approach to infectious disease is an essential aspect of modern health care. Viruses, in particular, play a big role.

This chapter examines the HIV/AIDS saga specifically, as it serves as a foundation for the coming chapters that look at infectious diseases and viruses even more broadly. I will discuss many anomalies here—including those relating to diagnoses, treatments, and transmissibility. The emerging narrative around HIV/AIDS is both troubling and eye-opening.

HIV/AIDS Background

According to the World Health Organization (WHO), "Human immunodeficiency virus (HIV) is an infection that attacks the body's immune system. Acquired immunodeficiency syndrome (AIDS) is the most advanced stage of the disease. HIV targets the body's white blood cells, weakening the immune system.... HIV is spread from the body fluids of an infected person, including blood, breast milk, semen and vaginal fluids."[1] Additionally, the WHO reports that 40.4 million people have died because of HIV, and, as of 2022, roughly 39 million people were living with HIV.[2] Author Joan Shenton summarizes the severity of the situation:

"The inexorable death sentence—'you have ten years at most' pronounced by doctors on young men and women has led to some of the most intense human suffering imaginable. **It has broken up families, alienated individuals from their communities, and led to psychological death and suicide."[3]** [emphasis added]

The condition was first reported in 1981 and caused an incredible panic. In 1984, Margaret Heckler, the Secretary of Health and Human Services, famously announced: "The probable cause of AIDS has been found," thanks to the work of Robert Gallo of the National Cancer Institute. It was a type of virus (specifically, a retrovirus), later named HIV. Author Celia Farber reports, "By the next day [the word] 'probable' had fallen away, and...HIV became forever lodged in global consciousness as 'the AIDS virus.'" Farber adds that "the word 'probable' was dropped when Lawrence Altman, writing in the *New York Times*, definitively referred to the retrovirus as 'the AIDS virus.' Altman, the *Times'* chief medical reporter, was at that time a member of a subdivision of the CDC called the Epidemic Intelligence Service (EIS), known as the 'medical CIA.'"[4]

However, Dr. Mikulas Popovic, one of the project researchers on Dr. Gallo's team, kept a duplicate of Dr. Gallo's original typewritten paper on HIV (originally referred to as HTLV-III). The document revealed that Dr. Gallo made key changes to the manuscript before submitting it to *Science*. In particular, he deleted Dr. Popovic's statement that **"despite intensive research efforts, the causative agent of AIDS has not yet been identified."** Dr. Gallo replaced it with the following sentence: "That a retrovirus of the HTLV family might be an etiologic agent of AIDS was suggested by the findings."[5] According to the Office of Research Integrity before the US Department of Health and Human Services: **"Dr. Gallo systematically rewrote the manuscript."[6]** [emphasis added]

The history-altering announcement in 1984 was made on the basis of Dr. Gallo's revised statement, and from then on, the medical establishment's position has been that HIV causes AIDS. The 2008 Nobel Prize in medicine was even awarded to Luc Montagnier, a French virologist, for co-discovering HIV.[7]

As Farber puts it, "On any given story, a dominant narrative takes shape, and journalists form a herd around it."[8] The HIV-AIDS connection has been one of those stories.

Does HIV=AIDS?

In spite of the apparent consensus portrayed by leading health organizations, many respected scientists disagreed, and currently disagree, with the narrative. **The specific point of controversy is *not* about whether people have been getting sick and dying. Instead, it is about whether HIV, specifically, is the *cause* of AIDS. Recall from the introduction: there are many potential causes to consider when people get sick, other than germs.**

The most notorious figure in this contrarian camp has been Peter Duesberg, PhD, a highly respected professor of molecular and cell biology at the University of California, Berkeley. As Farber reports: **"The cadre of scientists who signed a petition in 1991 stating they agreed with Duesberg...included three Nobel Laureates and 600 PhDs."**[9] [emphasis added]

One often-questioned aspect of the HIV-AIDS connection is the strange categorization of illness. Dr. Duesberg notes that a positive HIV test can suddenly recategorize an otherwise common illness, and HIV is "blamed." For example, if someone has tuberculosis *without* an HIV-positive test, then the person is diagnosed with tuberculosis, whereas if the person has tuberculosis *with* a positive HIV test, then the diagnosis is AIDS.[10]

Furthermore, Nancy Turner Banks, MD, a graduate of Harvard Medical School, views AIDS to be an "illusion of a new disease" that actually reflects "the cumulative massive intake of environmental pollutants, of toxic drugs, both legal and illegal, and the unprecedented stressor accumulation of modern life." She adds, "However, AIDS is not a disease; it is a syndrome—a collection of twenty-nine old diseases, clustered together, re-branded, and given a new scary label. It is a product marketed by fear, deception, and the creation of mass hysteria. It has been selling well for...years."[11]

In their book *Virus Mania* (2021), Torsten Engelbrecht; Claus Köhnlein, MD; Samantha Bailey, MD; and Stefano Scoglio, PhD, BSc, make a similar claim. They note that the definition of AIDS is "anything but coherent" because there is "no universal definition," and it can be diagnosed on the basis of "common and non-specific symptoms."[12]

Even Kary Mullis, the winner of the 1993 Nobel Prize in chemistry, vocally weighed in. In his book *Dancing Naked in the Mind Field* (1998), he wrote: "The CDC continues to add new diseases to the grand AIDS definition. The CDC has virtually doctored the books to make it appear as if the disease continues to spread."[13]

Beyond the issues around definitions and categorization, there are many other reasons why smart people challenge the "HIV-causes-AIDS" hypothesis. Dr. Mullis detailed his journey, and what he said was startling—particularly coming from a Nobel laureate:

> When I first heard in 1984 that [Montagnier and Gallo] had independently discovered that the retrovirus HIV...caused AIDS, I accepted it as just another scientific fact....
>
> Four years later I was working as a consultant at Specialty Labs in Santa Monica. Specialty was trying to develop a means of using [polymerase chain reaction (PCR)] to detect retroviruses in the thousands of blood donations received per day by the Red Cross. I was writing a report on our progress to our project sponsor, and I began by stating, "HIV is the probable cause of AIDS."
>
> I asked a virologist at Specialty where I could find the reference for HIV being the cause of AIDS.
>
> "You don't need a reference," he told me. "Everyone knows it."
>
> "I'd like to quote a reference." I felt a little funny about not knowing the source of such an important discovery. Everyone else seemed to.

"Why don't you cite the CDC report?" he suggested, giving me a copy of the Centers for Disease Control's periodic report on morbidity and mortality. I read it. It wasn't a scientific article. It simply said that an organism had been identified—it did not say how....The report did not identify the original scientific work, but that didn't surprise me. It was intended for physicians, who didn't need to know the source of the information. **Physicians assumed that if the CDC was convinced, there must exist real proof somewhere that HIV was the cause of AIDS....**

I did computer searches. Neither Montagnier, Gallo, nor anyone else had published papers describing experiments which led to the conclusion that HIV probably caused AIDS. I read the papers in *Science* for which they had become well known as AIDS doctors, but all they had said there was that they had found evidence of past infection by something which was probably HIV in some AIDS patients. **They found antibodies. Antibodies to viruses had always been considered evidence of past disease, not present disease. [That is, antibodies indicated that] the patient had saved himself. There was no indication in these papers that this virus caused a disease. They didn't show that everybody with the antibodies had the disease. In fact, they found some healthy people with antibodies....**

I finally had the opportunity to ask Dr. Montagnier about the reference when he lectured in San Diego at the grand opening of the UCSD AIDS Research Center....In response, Dr. Montagnier suggested, "Why don't you read the CDC report?"

"I read it," I said. "That doesn't really address the issue of whether or not HIV is the probable cause of AIDS, does it?"

He agreed with me. It was damned irritating. If Montagnier [who eventually won a Nobel Prize for

> co-discovering HIV] didn't know the answer, who the hell did?[14] [emphasis added]

Dr. Mullis began to realize what was happening when he stumbled across the work of Dr. Duesberg: "One night, I was driving from Berkeley to La Jolla, and I heard an interview on National Public Radio with Peter Duesberg, a prominent virologist in Berkeley. I finally understood why I was having so much trouble finding references that linked HIV to AIDS. There weren't any, Duesberg said. No one had ever proved that HIV causes AIDS."

However, once Dr. Duesberg challenged the establishment's position about HIV and AIDS, he faced serious consequences. As Dr. Mullis put it: "[When] Duesberg pointed out wisely from the sidelines...that there was no good evidence implicating [HIV], he was ignored. Editors rejected his manuscripts and committees of his colleagues began to question his need for having his research funds continued....He was [eventually] cut off from research funds. Thus disarmed, he was less of a threat to the growing AIDS establishment. He would not be invited back to speak at meetings of his former colleagues."[15]

Even though he was ostracized, Dr. Duesberg continued to challenge the "HIV=AIDS" narrative by presenting important anomalies. For instance, as recalled by Joan Shenton: "In September 1992, Duesberg's letter in *Science* drew attention to more than 800 documented US and European clinically diagnosed HIV-free AIDS cases, and upward of 2,200 in Africa that all met the WHO definition of AIDS. There may be more, said Duesberg, and [he] pointed out that only 50 percent of all AIDS cases reported by the CDC had been tested for HIV, with diagnoses [of untested individuals] based on their disease symptoms alone. Of those that *were* tested, 5 percent never showed signs of HIV."[16] Even Dr. Montagnier admitted, "It's quite possible that some other agent sometimes introduces some kind of autoimmune reaction that destroys the immune system. HIV is not the only one."[17]

Dr. Montagnier's reasoning, though somewhat open-minded, was still limited to allopathic-centric thinking. Maybe the issue wasn't just a biological "agent," as he alluded to, but lifestyle factors pertaining to overall health. Along these lines, Shenton and Celia Farber visited a village in Uganda—a part of the world that was allegedly an epicenter of AIDS. **They were told by local charity workers, "It's not so much AIDS, it's the fact that people here just don't have enough to eat. They are dying of malnutrition."**[18] [emphasis added]

Health problems in Africa weren't new, however. Dr. Harvey Bialy—who had worked for many years as a tropical-disease expert and was the scientific editor of *Bio/Technology*—stated in a 1988 interview: "I had thought for a long time that what was being classified as AIDS in Africa was a completely different syndrome of diseases than what was being called AIDS in the West. [It] was in fact nothing more than a new name for a collection of old diseases. Diseases that are called AIDS are classical African diseases in populations that have for a very long time been subject to these infections."[19] Separately, he added: **"From both my literature review and my personal experience over most of the so-called AIDS centres in Africa, I can find no believable persuasive evidence that Africa is in the midst of a new epidemic of infectious immunodeficiency."**[20] [emphasis added]

Furthermore, the diagnostic process around HIV/AIDS was sloppy. As Shenton writes: "The vast majority of AIDS cases in Africa were not diagnosed with HIV tests; these were too expensive for general use. AIDS was...diagnosed through the guidelines laid down by the WHO's Bangui clinical case definition. That is, they were not actually tested for HIV but were diagnosed positive or negative on the basis of a combination of symptoms. **This is called presumptive diagnosis. The trouble was that the combination of symptoms required for an AIDS diagnosis (prolonged fever, diarrhea, dry cough) were indistinguishable from those of old established diseases like tuberculosis and malaria."**[21] [emphasis added]

But, as Dr. Duesberg had warned, even when HIV tests are used, the results aren't always reliable. In fact, Dr. Banks begins her book *AIDS, Opium, Diamonds, and Empire* (2010) with a list of more than sixty factors that are known to cause false-positive HIV antibody test results. Among them are renal (kidney) failure, tuberculosis, flu, flu vaccination, tetanus vaccination, malaria, hemophilia, and pregnancy (in women who have given birth multiple times). As Dr. Banks sums up the situation, "The antibody tests supposedly detect antibodies against what are claimed to be HIV proteins or antigens.... **[However,] the proteins in the antibody test are cellular in origin and are not specific to HIV.**"[22] In other words, the tests are unreliable: they can show a positive result when in fact the test is picking up something unrelated to HIV.

Dr. Mullis, the inventor of another type of HIV-diagnostic test, PCR, even stated: **"With PCR, if you do it well, you can find almost anything in anybody....It doesn't tell you that you're sick, and it doesn't tell you that the thing you ended up with really was going to hurt you."**[23] [emphasis added]

In other words, the diagnostic tools are *indirect methods* that are used to claim that someone has the disease. Thus, their results can lead to incorrect conclusions. **This is critical—not just for HIV/AIDS, but for all indirect testing methods used in the field of medicine.**

The outcomes have been tragic. Consider the case of Hector Serverino in the Dominican Republic, who tested positive for HIV after a motorcycle accident and was refused surgery. His wife was in such terror that she committed suicide. Serverino later tested negative (twice) and lived a healthy life thereafter.[24] Shenton describes another case of a man who tested positive for HIV in 1986 and was then "treated like a leper." His dentist wore a helmet and a visor when treating him. The man was so afraid that he would infect others that he repeatedly washed his hands with bleach until they were raw. The man retested himself in 1991 and got a negative result. And he retested the sample that had shown a positive result in 1986, and it was now negative.[25] Additionally, Shenton ran a controlled experiment with HIV-positive participants and again found a lack of reliability. One man who had tested positive three times tested negative twice.[26]

Drug Use and HIV/AIDS in America

As has been suggested about HIV/AIDS cases in Africa, poor health/lifestyles might have also been the culprits of the disease in the United States—but for different reasons. Robert F. Kennedy Jr. notes in his bestselling book *The Real Anthony Fauci* (2021) that the first American AIDS patients were five gay men who were living a "fast lane" lifestyle that included recreational drugs and heavy antibiotic use (to treat conditions such as syphilis, gonorrhea, and hepatitis B).[27] More specifically, as written by Dr. Duesberg, early AIDS patients were also users of *poppers*, which refers to "the volatile nitrite liquid that had become the rage in the homosexual community for its ability to facilitate anal intercourse, as well as to maintain erections and prolong orgasms."[28] Kennedy elaborates on the use of poppers, which emerged in the wake of the sexual liberation movement:

> Poppers became a mainstay of the gay social scene in the late 1970s....Every porn shop, bar, and bathhouse locker room sold poppers....The saloons and dance halls reeked of their pungent chemical aroma. At the end of each evening, bartenders routinely announced, "Last call for alcohol, last call for poppers." Researchers believe poppers to be the direct cause of Kaposi's sarcoma, a rare form of skin cancer that afflicts the nose, throat, lungs, and skin. Kaposi's sarcoma was the initial disease indicator of AIDS, but it was also common in gay men who were not infected with HIV.
>
> Poppers can severely damage the immune system, genes, lungs, liver, heart, or the brain; they can produce neural damage similar to that of multiple sclerosis, [and] can have carcinogenic effects....
>
> Government researchers and regulatory officials supported the association [between the use of poppers and AIDS]. Prior to Gallo's announcement [that HIV probably causes AIDS], the CDC had targeted poppers as the likely culprit for AIDS.[29]

Furthermore, Professor David Durack, who served on the NIH's Bioethics Committee, comments that aside from drug-using homosexuals, the only other AIDS patients were "junkies." The excessive drug use was not good for their health.[30] Engelbrecht et al. also note in *Virus Mania* that the percentage of AIDS patients who are drug users is likely higher than is typically acknowledged:

> The CDC purposely skewed their statistics. Their weekly bulletins divided AIDS patients into groups (homosexuals, intravenous drug users, racial minorities, hemophiliacs), yet they attributed a lower percentage to junkies than homosexuals....This gave the impression that drug users were a less significant group among AIDS patients.
>
> The CDC only admitted they played with the numbers to those who meticulously probed for more information. Journalist and Harvard-educated analyst John Lauritsen discovered that 25 percent of AIDS patients statistically labeled homosexual were also drug users. But the CDC simply lumped all of these gay drug addicts into the homosexual category. For this reason, the portion of drug users was officially 17 percent, whereas in reality it should have been 35 percent (that is, more than one in three AIDS patients fits into the intravenous drug category).[31]

The fact that AIDS seems to preferentially impact certain demographics is also telling. Engelbrecht et al. note that in wealthy countries like the United States and Germany, "almost all AIDS patients are men who lead a self-destructive lifestyle with toxic drugs, medications, etc. In contrast, the official statistics say [the following about]...poor countries: A much larger proportion of the population has AIDS. Men and women are equally affected. Primarily, malnourished people suffer from AIDS."[32] Furthermore, the authors point out that "such a pathogen would inevitably have to attack all people in all countries of the world equally: men and women, straight and gay, African and European—and not, as statistics reveal, in a racial and gender-biased way, attacking certain populations at different rates."[33]

Toxic AIDS Treatments

Making matters worse, the AIDS treatments themselves are more toxic than is often acknowledged. In fact, poisonous medication was arguably responsible (at least in part) for the acceleration of the HIV-AIDS panic of the 1980s—because the deaths were attributed to AIDS rather than the medicine that was making people so sick.

A noteworthy story from 1985 is the death of Rock Hudson, who was one of the first known celebrities to die from AIDS. In 2020, *Men's Health* even noted that Hudson "changed the AIDS movement."[34] Actress Morgan Fairchild said that "Rock Hudson's death gave AIDS a face."[35] His death initiated massive fundraising for AIDS research, including support from actress Elizabeth Taylor.

Hudson was bisexual, and one of his lovers reported that Hudson had offered him poppers. He was also a heavy drinker and smoker and had quadruple bypass surgery. Although he appeared to be unhealthy by his own devices, his AIDS medication might have pushed him over the edge. He took a drug called HPA-23, which has liver-destroying effects. According to William Haseltine of Harvard Medical School, the drug hadn't been tested with properly controlled scientific studies to evaluate its safety and efficacy. He called it a "crime."[36]

But Hudson's death wasn't marketed as something related to a poor lifestyle or a poisonous drug. Rather, the messaging was that a deadly virus led to his demise.

In 1988, an AIDS treatment drug called AZT was announced.[37] Anthony Fauci, MD, the director of the National Institute of Allergy and Infectious Diseases, stated in an interview: "The reason that only one drug has been made available, AZT, [is] because it's the only drug that has thus far been shown, in scientifically controlled trials, to be safe and effective."[38]

The medication was developed in the 1960s to kill cancer cells (that is, it was an old chemotherapy drug). Engelbrecht et al. note that when AZT's inventor ran studies on test mice, they all died "from the extreme toxicities of AZT."[39] Dr. Duesberg concurred, stating that "AZT is definitely toxic, indiscriminately killing virus-infected and uninfected T-cells alike."[40] In fact, AZT's inventor didn't think to patent the drug because it was "so worthless."[41] Even the head of the FDA worried that approving the drug would represent a "significant and potentially dangerous departure from our normal toxicology requirements."[42]

AZT's release as an AIDS drug was based on a 1987 study that has been criticized, because (among other problems) the experiments stopped after four months. That means longer-term side effects remained unstudied.[43] However, after four years, 80 percent of the study's participants had died, and shortly thereafter, all of them were dead.[44] Furthermore, a lengthy 1993 study of AZT—the first one *not* funded by the maker of the drug—revealed that AZT was, in fact, shortening lives.[45]

To Dr. Banks, there is no question about what was happening. She remarks: "Clearly, AZT causes AIDS. When patients begin to deteriorate...they are told that the *HIV* has developed immunity to the drug and that the HIV is killing them, when, in fact, it is the drug, AZT."[46]

Professional tennis player Arthur Ashe, who died from AIDS, had been taking high doses of AZT.[47] Ashe acknowledged in the *Washington Post* in 1992, "The confusion for AIDS patients like me is that there is a growing school of thought that HIV may not be the sole cause of AIDS, and the standard treatments such as AZT actually make matters worse." He apparently wanted to stop taking AZT but asked the *New York Daily News*, "What will I tell my doctors?"[48]

Professional basketball player Magic Johnson, who is still alive as of 2023, has a different story. Dr. Duesberg explains it in his book *Inventing the AIDS Virus* (1996):

> In November 1991, Magic proved to be HIV-positive when he applied for a marriage license. Magic was totally healthy until...[doctors] advised AIDS prophylaxis with AZT. Magic's health changed radically within a few days. The press wrote in December 1991: "Magic Reeling as Worst Nightmare Comes True—He's Getting Sicker." Only after he began taking AZT did Magic's health begin to decline. He "had lost his appetite and suffered from bouts of nausea and fatigue" and complained, "I feel like vomiting almost every day."
>
> But then suddenly Magic's AIDS symptoms disappeared—and so did all further news about his AIDS symptoms and treatment. Had Magic's virus suddenly become harmless, or was Magic taken off AZT? No paper would mention whether Magic was taken off AZT. Nobody knew, except those who joked, "There is no magic in AZT, and there is no AZT in Magic." Indeed, it is very unlikely that he could have won the Olympics in 1992 on AZT, considering his strong reactions to the toxic drug in 1991. The silence of the AIDS establishment seems to confirm this assumption. Nothing would have been a better advertisement for the troubled AIDS drug than having returned AIDS patient Magic to an Olympic victory. But no such announcement was made. At last Magic broke the silence himself. After a "motivational" AIDS talk in Tallahassee, Florida, in the spring of 1995, Magic responded to a teacher that he had been "taking AZT for a while," but had "stopped." The media preferred not to mention the news.[49]

Shenton and her team also investigated AZT. They sought out long-term HIV survivors by placing advertisements in gay-focused newspapers and magazines, and indeed found a number of long-term survivors, many of whom had been HIV-positive for more than ten years. **Shenton writes: "The one thing the long-term survivors had in common was that they had refused to take AZT from the very beginning. Several of them said they had seen**

friends die who went on AZT and continued with their drug-taking habits."[50] [emphasis added]

But, as Engelbrecht et al. note, there was so much fear about AIDS that many doctors "refused to make any connection with the highly toxic antiviral AZT. Their belief in the deadliness of HIV was so firm that they weren't even shocked when all patients died within a short time."[51] (Note: Further details about the sordid AZT saga are illuminated in John Lauritsen's book *Poison by Prescription: The AZT Story* [1990].)

Engelbrecht and his colleagues mention that in 1993, AIDS case rates in the US "doubled overnight" because of a redefinition of AIDS: a positive HIV test accompanied by certain levels of CD4 cells automatically constituted an "AIDS" diagnosis.[52] The authors continue: "The broadening of the AIDS definition meant that many people had the 'AIDS patient' label superimposed on them, even though they were actually not sick at all."[53] **But in the mid-1990s, *death* rates started to decline. Engelbrecht et al. note that part of this might have been due to "the drastic reductions in doses of AIDS drugs like AZT."[54]** [emphasis added]

HIV/AIDS Contagion Anomalies

Another perplexing feature of HIV/AIDS is that there are instances of failed transmission. One often-cited work by HIV/AIDS contrarians is a ten-year prospective study published in the *American Journal of Epidemiology* in 1997 by Nancy Padian, PhD, et al.[55] Dr. Banks writes: "[Padian et al.'s] findings have turned the AIDS establishment into defensive name calling and sputtering idiocy in their attempt to reinterpret the findings from this well-designed study. The long-term prospective study provides no evidence that HIV is sexually transmitted....The Padian group found that the efficiency of HIV is so low by sexual means that one must find another reason to question why any HIV test is positive."[56] David Rasnick, PhD, concurred with this interpretation of the study in his detailed 2003 letter to the *BMJ*, citing a number of other works that challenge the HIV transmission hypothesis.[57]

However, defenders of the mainstream HIV/AIDS narrative assert that such claims reflect misinterpretations of the study.[58]

Outside the controversy over that study, others have reported transmission anomalies. Shenton writes: "Bill Paxton, a Scottish immunologist working in New York, has found that several high-risk but uninfected people had blood cells that could not be infected with HIV, no matter how many doses of virus was added to their blood."[59] The same thing happened with a thirty-nine-year-old gay man, who previously had "years of promiscuity." He underwent "repeated attempts…to infect his blood in vitro with HIV but without success."[60] Similarly, Shenton mentions "the wife of a hemophiliac who has remained uninfected although she had unprotected sex with her HIV-positive husband for two years before he realized he 'had the disease.'"[61]

Robert Willner, MD, PhD, even injected himself—on multiple occasions—with a needle that had been dipped in the blood of an allegedly HIV-infected individual. He didn't get HIV. A video of one such instance from 1994 is still available online (including the press conference he held around the event).[62]

Finally, Dr. Duesberg reported on anomalies in Africa with prostitutes—and more—in his 1996 book:

> To a large extent, the myth of an African AIDS epidemic grew out of a report in the late 1980s entitled *Voyage des Krynen en Tanzanie*. Written by French charity workers Philippe and Evelyne Krynen, it dramatically summarized their findings of devastated villages, abandoned homes, growing numbers of orphans, and a sexually transmitted AIDS epidemic that threatened to depopulate the Kagera province of northern Tanzania. As the heads of Partage, the largest AIDS charity for Tanzanian children, the Krynens told a story that the news media could not resist, one that is still repeated today. The vivid images helped shape the Western impression of an AIDS problem out of control.

> But after spending a few years working with the people of the Kagera, the Krynens changed their minds. To their own disbelief, they discovered no AIDS epidemic in the region at all. **The "sexually transmitted" disease somehow completely missed the prostitutes while it killed their clients; the exact same prostitutes work the towns today. Whatever caused AIDS in these clients did not affect these hardy prostitutes.** Then the Krynens discovered that more than half their "AIDS" patients tested negative for HIV. The empty houses turned out to be additional homes owned by Tanzanians who had moved to the city. And the final blow came from the "orphans" themselves, who turned out to be the consequences of the Tanzanian social structure; the parents typically moved to the cities to earn money, leaving the grandparents to care for the children. "There is no AIDS," Philippe Krynen now states flatly. "It is something that has been invented. There are no epidemiological grounds for it; it doesn't exist for us."[63] [emphasis added]

Weaponizing Disease

Shenton summarizes the contrarian HIV/AIDS position well: "None of the established principles about HIV and AIDS have stood up to the test. There has been no heterosexual pandemic; AIDS has remained firmly locked into the high-risk groups; AIDS has not behaved like a sexually transmitted disease should, and no cure for AIDS has been found."[64]

One might then wonder: Given the many anomalies, can all of the blame be placed on ignorance? Or was there an orchestration by powerful people who pulled the strings at key moments, and well-meaning individuals just fell for it?

In the opinion of Dr. Banks: "AIDS was created to cover both… the toxic poisoning of young people in the West and the industrial poisoning and social disruption in Africa. It was pure insanity, but it worked….Because allopathic physicians are trained in recognizing and treating the infectious problems of the 19th century, the 20th-century problem of systemic toxicity was misdiagnosed."[65] She continues, "HIV fit perfectly into the war model of social organization at the foundation of Western civilization.... Allopathic medicine as a fundamental part of that system logically conspires. The virus was the enemy."[66]

Additionally, in Robert F. Kennedy Jr.'s book *The Real Anthony Fauci*, he refers to the HIV/AIDS crisis as a "template" that was used again with COVID-19.[67]

Whatever forces might be behind HIV/AIDS, it has caused a significant amount of damage to people's lives all over the world. It demonstrates clearly the way in which modern medicine can be weaponized in order to terrorize the global population. And it was all possible because of the belief in a contagious virus that causes a deadly disease. Therefore, in order to see through potential future fiascos, and to up our game in terms of our understanding of health and disease, it's essential to double-click on what viruses are and how they're studied. This is a critical exercise in the process of unwinding allopathic medicine's stronghold over modern thinking.

CHAPTER 2

VIRUS ISOLATION

In the previous chapter, the HIV/AIDS crisis was presented as a struggle between two battling perspectives: one that believed the mainstream narrative claiming "HIV causes AIDS," and the other that disagreed. This is a relatively well-known split. However, what is less-often discussed is a divide *within* the crowd of dissenters. Among those who believed that HIV does not cause AIDS, a small minority argued that *HIV does not exist*. In other words, this minority acknowledged that the researchers who claimed to have discovered HIV were indeed mixing things in test tubes and taking pictures of what appeared under microscopes. But in all of that work, they never found an isolated, purified virus. Rather, they were working with a "soup" of cellular material that they simply *assumed* contained the virus within it. Going forward, I will refer to those who espouse this perspective as the "No Virus" camp.

The Perth Group in Australia conducted extensive analyses on this matter and even published peer-reviewed papers. The group also produced a detailed (and lengthy) scientific paper that critiques the foundational HIV studies, titled "HIV—a virus like no other" (it is available for free at http://www.theperthgroup.com/). Neville Hodgkinson, formerly a medical and science correspondent of the London *Daily Mail* and the *Sunday Times*, has published many articles about the Perth Group's work, including a summary of its six key assertions.[1]

Additionally, a German virologist named Stefan Lanka was vocal about the No Virus position during the HIV/AIDS era and continues to be today.[2] In a 2021 interview, Dr. Lanka comments:

> What I saw in both papers—of [Drs.] Gallo and Montagnier—...they claim[ed] a virus, but they never *saw* a virus....[In their work], only an enzymatic activity [indicated to them] that there *should be* a virus somewhere else around....As the cells [in the experiments] were dying, they [thought] that...at least some of the materials...are viral. It's their secret how they could choose some of them and say, "Look, those are the viral proteins," using the antibody test....When I realized that there is a virus in the title [of the paper] but no virus structure inside, I thought I [must] have over[looked] something. Or medical doctors are keeping their real isolation protocol secret....I was not speaking with anybody on this because I was afraid [of] losing my lab.[3]

He then started looking into other viruses, not just HIV, and the same methodological problems were there. He's been open about his critiques of the field of virology ever since.[4]

Nancy Turner Banks, MD, a Harvard-trained doctor, was also explicit in her book *AIDS, Opium, Diamonds, and Empire* (2010), arguing that Dr. Robert Gallo only described "indirect surrogate markers" in his HIV work in the early 1980s.[5] **She further explained that isolation of the virus was "never done" by Dr. Gallo or Nobel Prize winner Luc Montagnier. Dr. Banks cites a 1997 interview in which Dr. Montagnier admitted that in his 1983 experiment, "we saw some particles, but they did not have the morphology typical of retroviruses....I repeat, we did not purify.**"[6] The magnitude of this statement should not be underestimated. [emphasis added]

However, Dr. Peter Duesberg—perhaps the most famous of the HIV-causes-AIDS dissenters—strongly disagreed with the

No Virus view. He called the divide over the existence of the virus "tragic."[7] Henry Bauer, a professor emeritus of chemistry and science studies at Virginia Tech, addressed this issue in the foreword he wrote to the 2014 edition of Joan Shenton's book *Positively False: Exposing the Myths Around HIV and AIDS*. **He wrote: "Since [the] distraction has become an open, unpleasant, regrettable schism, it would nowadays warrant extended and explicit analysis."[8]** [emphasis added]

Dr. Bauer foreshadowed what happened with SARS-CoV-2 beginning in 2020 and continues today in 2023 as I am writing this book. The same arguments that were made to refute the existence of HIV are being made about the methods used to isolate and purify SARS-CoV-2...*and every other virus claimed to exist*. Yes, you read that correctly. They say that viruses do not exist. (Note: In case you're wondering, the No Virus position does not deny the existence of bacteria. However, as will be discussed in chapter 3, the No Virus position views bacteria as part of the body's internal cleanup crew rather than pathogenic instigators.)

Also, to be clear, the No Virus camp isn't denying that people get sick. Rather, the claim is that people get sick for a multitude of reasons other than alleged intracellular parasites known as "viruses." Yet, the allopathic model is often so focused on germs that it misses important factors that impact health.

This may be causing significant confusion and disbelief in your mind.

But consider, for example, that New Zealand's Institute of Environmental Science and Research (ESR)—which claims to have isolated SARS-CoV-2 and sequenced its genome—responded on July 19, 2022, to an Official Information Act request with the following statement: "ESR has not performed any experiments to scientifically prove the existence of SARS-CoV-2 virus and therefore not [*sic*] provide you with any records."[9] The request had asked for "all records in the possession, custody, or control of the ESR that scientifically proves the existence of SARS-CoV-2" (and went on to clarify that the

experiments should follow the scientific method, demonstrate repeatability, and use proper controls).[10]

Whether the virus *causes* the COVID-19 illness was also questioned in a separate request. On August 17, 2022, New Zealand's ESR responded as follows: "ESR has not performed any experiments to scientifically prove that [the] SARS-CoV-2 virus causes COVID-19 and therefore not [*sic*] provide you with any records."[11] The request had asked for "all records in the possession, custody, or control of the ESR that scientifically proves SARS-CoV-2 virus causes COVID-19 disease" (and went on to clarify that the experiments should follow the scientific method, demonstrate repeatability, and use proper controls).[12]

But it's not just New Zealand.

The CDC's November 2, 2020, response to a request for "all records in the possession, custody or control of the CDC describing the isolation of the SARS-COV-2 virus" was met with the following response: "A search of our records failed to reveal any documents pertaining to your request."[13]

This is just a snapshot of more than 200 organizations in forty countries that have failed to provide evidence along similar lines. And the No Virus position has had favorable rulings in German courts (more on these topics later in this chapter). [all emphasis in the quotes above were added]

So what does the No Virus group think has been happening over the past several years with COVID-19?[14] This relates to a deeper question about which allopathic medicine often lacks an understanding: *Why do people get sick?*[15] Answering that question is a distinct exercise from determining whether SARS-CoV-2 exists in the first place (and second, if it does exist, whether it causes disease). The No Virus argument is more focused on the question of the existence of the virus itself. Having a definitive alternative explanation for disease is not required to refute the existence of SARS-CoV-2.

However, since you, the reader, are likely wondering what's going on, what follows is a set of possibilities—as an exercise in critical thinking—but nothing definitive. **It's important to first repeat something basic in an effort to alleviate inevitable psychological hurdles: people in the same place, around the same time, can get sick with similar symptoms because of many factors that have nothing to do with viruses.** Put another way, it can't be assumed that a contagious virus is what causes illness simply because people went to a party and a lot of them got sick. For instance, in chapter 1, I discussed a number of possibilities with regard to the symptoms associated with the label "HIV/AIDS"—people got sick because of toxicity, drug use, unhealthy lifestyles, harmful medications, malnutrition, and more.

There are countless factors that can contribute to illness, more generally. In the modern world, we're bombarded with a sea of toxic substances in our food, water, air, medicines, homes, buildings, clothing fabrics, cosmetic products, sunscreens, deodorants, kitchen appliances, plastic containers, furniture, detergents, masks, motor fuel, metal can linings, soaps and shampoos, perfumes and colognes, air fresheners, insect repellents, toys, baby powders, dental procedures, and more.[16] **Certain locations might result in more exposure to these toxins than others, thereby causing concentrations of illness—and very specific symptoms—that have nothing to do with germs.** Seasonality can also play into illness, as there are changes in humidity, temperature, barometric pressure, and exposure to sunlight. Electric and magnetic fields (EMFs) are everywhere in the wireless era and are especially prevalent in certain places;[17] and electricity itself has become more widespread in our world, which might be more harmful than is often acknowledged.[18] Radiation exposure can cause people in the same location to get sick—which is what happened after the Chernobyl nuclear meltdown in 1986.

In fact, governments have a history of experimenting on their own people (such as the openly acknowledged MK-ULTRA mind-control program).[19] Colin Ross, MD, gives a relevant example of unethical experimentation in his book *The CIA Doctors: Human*

Rights Violations by American Psychiatrists (2006): "Clouds of radioactive material were released into the atmosphere and tracked as they moved downwind, often through populated areas" from 1948 to 1952 in Utah, Tennessee, New Mexico, and the state of Washington. Ross also references an initiative called GREEN RUN, which involved the release of radioactive iodine-131 in Washington, and the cloud "contained hundreds and perhaps thousands as times [*sic*] as much radiation as was released accidentally at Three Mile Island in 1979."[20] Along similar lines, Joe Biden's administration spoke openly in 2022 about considering "geoengineering" to block the sun because of "climate change." The *Daily Beast* notes: "This is a technique that essentially involves spraying fine aerosols into the atmosphere."[21] Unacknowledged radiation and/or toxic aerosols could cause people in the same place to get sick with similar symptoms around the same time—not a virus. This needs to be considered within a comprehensive and open-minded analysis.

Also, nutritional deficiencies can cause symptoms of severe illness that can be mistaken for contagion. Consider scurvy, a deadly condition that killed more than 2 million sailors at sea starting in the Christopher Columbus era.[22] Scurvy can cause exhaustion, the loss of teeth, ulcerations on the gums, spontaneous bleeding, limb pain, swelling, and anemia.[23] There were many sailors in the same place at the same time who got sick—with similar, specific symptoms—and died. The problem was solved when sailors started consuming foods with vitamin C. They weren't all sick, in the same place and at the same time, because of a contagious virus—all they needed to do was eat some lemons. Similarly, beriberi—a condition that affects the nerves, heart, digestion, and limbs—is now known to be caused by a deficiency of thiamine (vitamin B1)—not a contagious virus.[24] Another one is pellagra, a condition that causes skin lesions and neurological and gastrointestinal disturbances. It is now known to result from a deficiency in niacin (vitamin B3), not a contagious virus.[25]

Furthermore, an analysis of COVID-19, specifically, is complicated by the fact that multiple doses of a vaccine were introduced into the global population. This needs to be considered as a possible contributor to illness, as the vaccine's toxicity—in the short and long term—is not fully understood (more on this later). Most people don't even know the ingredients of the fluid that was injected into their body, let alone what the impacts on their health might be. And the analysis is even more muddled because of data problems arising from false-positive test results.[26] Also, some deaths were attributed to COVID-19 when the real cause of death was something else, and yet a COVID-19-positive test led to a "COVID-19-death" classification.[27] So it's difficult to ascertain accurate data about what actually happened.

Psychological factors, such as mass fear on a global scale, have also been significant, and might negatively affect health. This will become more pertinent later in the book when consciousness is discussed. Consider, as well, that female roommates' menstrual cycles sometimes synchronize, and that's not because of a contagious germ.[28] Might there even be an invisible resonance between people that mimics germ-based contagion but is not understood by modern science?

Additionally, there are often cases in which some people in the same place have gotten sick with "COVID-19" symptoms, and yet others *didn't*. If it's so contagious, shouldn't every single person get sick? These anomalies are not well explained beyond unproven theories or wild guesses. Such anomalies cannot be swept under the rug, but often they are.

Ultimately, there are so many considerations and possibilities—some of which people have thought of, and others that are perhaps beyond our current understanding of science and medicine. Scientists only know what 4 percent of the universe is made out of, and the rest—96 percent of the universe—is considered to be "dark matter" and "dark energy." **The true answer as to why people have gotten sick during the COVID-19 era—in contrast to reductionistic, allopathic thinking—might be *multifactorial*.[29]**

So, the No Virus position doesn't purport to know exactly *why* the symptoms associated with COVID-19 emerged *when* they did—but—to repeat—*not having a definitive explanation for symptoms doesn't prove that it was a virus.* "I don't know" is an acceptable answer sometimes, albeit unsatisfying. And it's better than getting stuck in an incorrect belief.

However, the No Virus position is about much more than SARS-CoV-2. And it's about much more than HIV/AIDS. **It is about challenging a scientific paradigm that is fundamental to allopathic medicine.**

The No Virus position further argues that flawed methodologies have been used by virologists since the inception of the field. That's why they claim that no virus has been shown to exist. For example, scientists claimed that viruses caused disease well before the technology existed that could see something so tiny. They just *assumed* that viruses were there. Also, the term *virus* used to mean "poison."[30]

From the No Virus perspective, the belief in disease-causing viruses is thus still a *hypothesis*—not an established scientific "theory." Therefore, the onus is on the modern scientific establishment to back up its claim that viruses exist and cause disease. It's as if scientists got ahead of themselves and ran with a belief system that's supposed to be accepted as fact, when in reality, the basics still need to be validated using the scientific method.

Additionally, the No Virus position does not intend to imply that the majority of hardworking scientists and doctors are willfully conspiring and lying—although it doesn't deny that *some* of them are intentionally bad actors. But this exercise is not about pointing fingers at individuals or trying to guess what their intentions are. In fact, the majority of well-meaning scientists and doctors are likely overlooking fundamental problems that are baked into the foundations of virology. Either they haven't thought to question what they were taught, or they're too afraid to challenge the establishment's positions because the implications would be too devastating for the entire field. And it could be devastating to their own careers to speak out against the establishment's positions. Therefore, it's easier to "go along to get along."

If it seems too difficult to believe that something so important could fool so many smart people, just think of the many Ponzi schemes that have successfully defrauded otherwise savvy investors.

The No Virus position also acknowledges that scientists in virology labs are doing research—and it's true that they're working with toxic substances—whether they label their work "gain of function,"[31] "bioweapons research," or something else. However, the exact nature of the microscopic stuff in the test tubes they're mixing might be different from what we're told. And scientists are certainly seeing *something* under a microscope—but seeing something under a microscope doesn't necessarily mean that it's a virus.

As COVID-19 has persisted, this debate has been heating up. Drs. Thomas Cowan, Andrew Kaufman, Samantha Bailey, Mark Bailey, and many others have been vocally criticizing virology and its methods, and they have amassed large followings as more people ask questions about the prevailing narrative. Dr. Mark Bailey's "A Farewell to Virology" (published in September 2022 and available for free at https://drsambailey.com/a-farewell-to-virology-expert-edition/) is a seminal, technical piece that critiques the foundational virology studies claiming to have isolated SARS-CoV-2 (and other viruses). Additionally, in mid-2023, a 150-plus-hour online library of videos that discuss the No Virus position, and additional topics, was launched by Alec Zeck, Mike Winner, and others. It is titled "The End of COVID" (available at https://theendofcovid.com/). It had more than 100,000 sign-ups in the first several weeks of its launch.[32] Dr. Samantha Bailey—who was formerly a health presenter on New Zealand national television—has also posted many videos that explain the No Virus perspective in an easy-to-understand manner (they are available for free at https://drsambailey.com/resources/). Mike Stone's https://ViroLIEgy.com also covers these topics in detail. And even prior to COVID-19, related concepts were presented in the comprehensive books *Virus Mania* (originally published in 2007 and updated in 2021) by Torsten Engelbrecht and his colleagues; and *What Really Makes You Ill?* (2019) by Dawn Lester and David Parker.

The point is, the No Virus movement is strong, and it's growing. It is also causing an acrimonious divide among members of the "health-freedom community" who otherwise vigorously challenge the allopathic model of medicine. The No Virus position "goes too far" for the majority of them, but their rebuttals often suggest that they haven't studied the rationale for the position. That is, many of them aren't even aware of what the No Virus position is truly claiming, or why.[33]

Since this is such a fundamental issue for science and medicine, it does indeed need to be addressed with an "extended and explicit analysis" (to use Dr. Bauer's prophetic words following the HIV-AIDS debates). The allopathic model and the massive industries surrounding it are heavily dependent on the belief in disease-causing viruses, and the No Virus position challenges its core. In fact, tyrannical "pandemic measures" are made possible by the belief in a microscopic, deadly, contagious virus.

Moreover, the nature of the No Virus arguments—and the analytical processes involved—have caused members of the No Virus community to rethink presuppositions about fields beyond virology, including the nature of the cell, the atom, DNA, and other related topics (many of which are being explored by researchers such as Dr. Cowan but are beyond the scope of this book).[34] **Thus, this exercise is ultimately even more important than just reexamining virology and allopathic medicine; it's a way of approaching *all* scientific questions in a logical and scientific manner.**

As a society, we need to get this right—one way or the other.

Therefore, what follows in this chapter is an attempt to characterize the No Virus position as it has been presented by its proponents—so that you, the reader, will at least know what the arguments are, regardless of whether they are deemed to be compelling. This chapter presents a mere synopsis of the key issues, and additional resources are provided in the endnotes and bibliography.

The "best case" scenario appears to be that virology has conducted sloppy "science" in many cases. The "worst case" scenario is that the entire field of virology is a house of cards.

The Basics of the No Virus Argument

The debate about the existence of viruses leads to an examination of inherently technical subjects. The matter simply cannot be resolved without looking at the virology studies themselves. **More specifically, the matter cannot be resolved without reading the methods section of the foundational studies. This is a critical distinction, because sometimes a paper's stated conclusion is not aligned with what actually happened in the study. If a paper says, "We isolated the virus" in its title, do we know for sure that this is actually the case?**

Although virology studies are filled with technical jargon, the *principles* to examine are actually quite basic. To simplify, the two primary methodological problems that No Virus advocates typically raise are as follows:

1. Viruses are not physically isolated in virology experiments, which means that viruses cannot be known to exist. In fact, virology experiments lack an independent variable and are thus not designed to be capable of scientifically studying a virus.[35]

2. Virology studies lack proper controls.

The failure to properly do these two things demonstrates that the field of virology does not follow the scientific method, thereby rendering it one of "pseudoscience."[36] That is the No Virus position.

On the first point—*isolation*—*Merriam-Webster* defines the word as follows: "to set apart from others."[37] Dr. Cowan often gives a basic example: if someone has a toolkit with a hammer, a screwdriver, nails, and other tools, the process of isolating the hammer would be to take the hammer out of the toolkit and separate it from the other tools. Sometimes the word *purify* is used interchangeably with *isolate* in virology (although the definitions can become points of contention depending on how the terms are used). **Nobel laureate Dr. Luc Montagnier expressed how important the isolation/purification step is when he said that its purpose is "to make sure you have a real virus."[38]** [emphasis added]

In studies that seek to determine whether a virus makes people sick, a scientist would want to isolate the virus and then introduce it into living systems. That way, a scientist would be able to determine the effect the virus is having. Pictures of the virus could then be taken with an electron microscope to confirm a purified specimen, and analyses could then be run on the virus's biochemical composition. A virus—by itself—must be isolated first (as is done with bacteria).

In such a study, the virus would be known as the "independent variable"—the thing that is being tested. The hypothesis of the study might be, for instance, that when an isolated virus is introduced into a group of cells, it damages them. **In order to test that hypothesis—and this is the critical point—the scientists would need to establish that *only* the virus is being introduced and not other cellular debris, organisms, and so forth.** If things other than the virus are introduced into the experiment, how would experimenters know if the virus, specifically, is causing the effect? More fundamentally, how would they even know that the virus exists if they haven't isolated it first? And furthermore, if they haven't found the virus first, how would they know if, say, the feared SARS-CoV-2 "spike protein" *comes from* a virus, or whether the genetic material found *comes from* a virus?

Think of it another way. Imagine that Jill drinks a green juice every day; and it's made from a combination of celery juice, kale juice, apple juice, and lemon juice. Every time she drinks it, she gets an upset stomach. In order to find out what is causing her upset stomach, what should she do?

She decides to run an experiment. She drinks each of the ingredients individually to determine if one of them causes her to get an upset stomach. She does so, and sure enough, when she drinks plain kale juice—with no other juices mixed in—she gets an upset stomach. The other juices don't cause any problems. In this process, she *isolated* the kale juice.

The No Virus position is that this isolation process is not properly done in virology studies—using the common definition of *isolation*.

Therefore, a virus is assumed to exist, but it is never identified *on its own*, and thus it cannot be known to exist with certainty. So the kale-juice example wasn't a perfect analogy. In that case, kale juice was identified as a separate entity that could be isolated, whereas in virology experiments, the hypothesized virus isn't actually isolated—it's just assumed to be there.

Most people, including doctors, have no idea that this is an issue because they've never evaluated virology studies themselves, so they assume virologists are doing their jobs properly.

The second core assertion of the No Virus position is that virology studies lack proper controls. This is, by definition, the case because without first having an independent variable, proper controls cannot be conducted.[39]

Consider the following hypothetical situation: Joe gets sick every time he drinks milk. That's the only thing he tells his doctor, so the doctor concludes: *I know what's happening. Joe has a milk allergy.*

Why is this observation—by itself—not sufficient to form the conclusion that the milk is causing Joe's sickness? Maybe *any* drink would cause Joe to get sick (because, perhaps, he has a problem in his digestive tract). The doctor could run a simple control experiment, whereby he tells Joe to drink a more inert substance, such as water. If Joe gets sick after drinking milk and not water, that would be a greater indicator that milk is the cause.

But that's not enough. What if an invisible, toxic chemical on the glass was causing Joe's sickness? In that case, maybe milk wouldn't have anything to do with Joe's sickness. The doctor could then tell Joe to drink milk from different glasses and instruct him to do the same with water. And he could also suggest to Joe that he should drink different brands of milk, in case his sickness was caused by one brand in particular.

But even that's not enough. The doctor might wonder if the *location* in which Joe drank the milk had high levels of environmental toxins, mold, and/or radiation. So he could instruct Joe to drink milk in an entirely different location.

Then he could ask Joe to drink milk at different times of the day, in case something about his body clock makes him more or less sensitive at different times. He might also wonder if Joe should try drinking milk before, during, and after meals—maybe the timing of drinking milk relative to eating food is playing a role.

There are countless variables that should be explored in truly scientific work.

The point is that simply observing something doesn't necessarily tell a scientist what is *causing* what. An observation is just an observation. Therefore, studies need to be conducted in order to eliminate variables that could confuse the results (known as *confounding variables*).

This backdrop provides a context with which to explore the field of virology.

Changing Definitions of a Virus

A simple—yet often overlooked—question is as follows: *How do we know that viruses exist and that they cause disease?* Dr. Thomas Cowan, who has been asking this very question, clarifies: "To be clear, I don't mean an answer such as 'You do a test for the virus,' or 'All doctors believe there is such a virus.' I am specifically referring to the steps any virologist in the world should take to identify a new virus....In a sane and rational world, medical authorities would have made the answer to this straightforward question the first and highest priority in their role as educators of the population."[40]

Even David Baltimore, PhD, a Nobel laureate for his work in virology,[41] didn't have a good answer to this question when he was asked in a documentary how he would isolate and photograph HIV. **His response was: "Didn't Dr. Gallo do that? I mean, he actually isolated it....I mean, why should I do all of this? This is all textbook stuff you're asking me....I don't want to be your textbook. I got other things to do."**[42] [emphasis added]

We're accustomed to turning on the news, or reading an article, and seeing an image of a structure that we're told is a virus. We're told that it's been genetically sequenced. End of story. At that point, as the thinking goes, there's no need to ask questions because people's lives are at stake, and we should simply "trust the science."

But in order to show that a virus exists, one first needs to know what a virus is. As noted in *A History of Experimental Virology* (1991) by Alfred Grafe: "Celsus [a first-century AD Roman medical writer]...summarized the teachings of Hippocrates and the Greek schools of medicine, which he had translated into Latin. He employed the word virus to mean the equivalent of the Greek poison ios....**[A virus was considered to be] a slimy poison of visible origin.** This is illustrated by the dog roaming with rage depicted in Egyptian, Greek, and Roman literature, as well as in the constellation of the dog star Sirius, where it unites man and the Gods."[43] [emphasis added]

Moreover, in the book *The Poisoned Needle*, published in 1957 by Eleanor McBean, PhD, she included definitions from the mid-20th century, and they demonstrate how varied opinions were:

> The 1940 Medical Dictionary defines virus as "the specific living principle by which an infectious disease is transmitted." The definition is vague and meaningless because there is no such thing as a "living" principle....
>
> The Scientific Encyclopedia says viruses have been obtained for experimentation by means of extremely powerful centrifuges which must be specially built. In the same article it is stated that viruses are so small that they cannot be seen by the most powerful microscopes. Then how do they know they produced any? Or is this game of *hide and seek* just another means of using up... millions of dollars?
>
> The Modern Encyclopedia (1944) says in part: "A *virus* differs from a *bacterium* in that the latter can live and reproduce itself in an artificial culture such as beef broth, whereas a virus must live inside a living cell....
>
> Webster's Dictionary refers to [a] *virus* as a "slimy or poisonous liquid."[44]

The modern definition of a virus is different today than it was in the past. As observed by virologist Dr. Stefan Lanka, the contemporary view of viruses was influenced by work on bacteriophages—viruslike entities found in pure bacteria cultures.[45] The 1969 Nobel Prize in medicine was awarded for work on bacteriophages dating back to the 1940s, and the final sentence of the Nobel Prize summary explains that this work **"is now generally accepted as the basic pattern of reproduction of *all* viruses."**[46] [emphasis added] (Note: While bacteriophages are sometimes regarded as agents that "infect" or "eat" bacteria, they have also been interpreted in a more benevolent light: they could be viewed as survival mechanisms for bacteria when they are in a stressed situation.[47])

Dr. Lanka also notes that James Watson and Francis Crick's 1953 paper published in *Nature* changed scientists' overall orientation. Watson and Crick's announcement of DNA's double-helix structure initiated the field of molecular biology, which examines the impact of genes on chemical processes within cells.[48] **As Dr. Lanka puts it: "From that moment on, the causes of disease were thought to be in the genes. The idea of a virus changed, and overnight a virus was no longer a toxin, but rather a dangerous genetic sequence, a dangerous DNA, a dangerous viral strand, etc. This new genetic virology was founded by young chemists who...had unlimited research money."**[49] [emphasis added]

As a result of these beliefs about bacteriophages and DNA, viruses in the modern era have taken on a specific definition that's different from past iterations. A summary definition is provided by a group of doctors, scientists, and researchers, as follows:

> [Viruses are] replicating, protein-coated pieces of genetic material, either DNA or RNA, [that] exist as independent entities in the real world and are able to act as pathogens. That is, the so-called particle with the protein coating and genetic interior is commonly believed to infect living tissues and cells, replicate inside these living tissues, damage the tissues as it makes its way out, and, in doing so, is also believed to create disease and sometimes death in its host—[this is] the

> so-called viral theory of disease causation. The alleged virus particles are then said to be able to transmit to other hosts, causing disease in them as well.[50]

First, it's noteworthy that the definition has changed so many times—and radically so. When people in past eras spoke of a "virus," they likely weren't describing the same thing that we're referring to today. Second, if we adopt the modern definition just described, one might wonder: *Has anyone ever seen such a microscopic thing performing all of those steps—infecting living tissues, replicating inside them, and then damaging cells on its way out?* A very specific set of steps needs to be validated in order to meet the modern definition of a virus. **A 2015 paper published in *PLOS Pathogens* doesn't inspire confidence: "How non-enveloped viruses penetrate a host membrane to enter cells and cause disease remains an enigmatic step."**[51] [emphasis added]

A Brief History of Germ Theory and Virology

The modern view of viruses posits not only that they exist, but that they *cause* disease in their host. This is a tenet of what's more generally called the "germ theory" of disease. Germ theory dominates contemporary allopathic thinking—not just regarding viruses but also bacteria and other microbes.

Germ theory wasn't always so prevalent, however. Edward Golub, a former Purdue University biology professor, noted: "Since the time of the ancient Greeks, people did not 'catch' a disease, they slipped into it. To catch something meant that there was something to catch....Most disease was due to deviation from a good life.... [And when diseases occurred] they could most often be set aright by changes in diet."[52]

In 1546, a Roman poet named Girolamo Fracastoro introduced a comprehensive germ-based theory that gained traction.[53] However, his theory came before the advent of the microscope, so the idea was highly theoretical. It wasn't until the 1670s that Antonie van Leeuwenhoek observed bacteria—but not viruses—under a microscope, which initiated the field of microbiology.[54] Bacteria are much larger than hypothesized viruses are believed to be.

Louis Pasteur *suspected* that a tiny virus existed through his work on rabies in the late 19th century, but he never saw a virus because the theorized particle was too small to be seen using the microscopes available at that time.[55] One wonders how he knew it was there if he didn't see it. In any event, Pasteur is a key figure, as he is widely credited for developing the germ theory of disease.[56] (Note: While Pasteur is regarded as a hero in allopathic medicine, in other circles he is vilified as a "plagiarist and impostor," while his contemporary Antoine Béchamp is lauded as a hero. This dynamic is explored in the book titled *Béchamp or Pasteur? A Lost Chapter in this History of Biology* by Ethel Hume [1923]. Also, historian Gerald Geison evaluated Pasteur's private notebooks, in a book published by Princeton University Press in 1995, and they revealed "sometimes astonishing...discrepancies between the results reported in [Pasteur's] published papers and those recorded in his private manuscripts."[57])

The electron microscope was invented in the 1930s, and it wasn't until this technology was available that anything as small as a hypothesized virus could be seen.[58] The first use of an electron microscope in clinical virology was around 1948, and commercial electron microscopes became widely available during the 1960s and 1970s.[59] **This is an important consideration: the ability to see virus-sized particles is a relatively new development.**

Yet, the first alleged discovery of a virus occurred decades before all of this. The Tobacco Mosaic Virus—a "virus" said to infect and damage tobacco and other plants—was described in Dmitri Ivanovsky's 1903 paper "Über die Mosaikkrankheit der Tabakspflanze" (About the Mosaic Disease of the Tobacco Plant).[60] This is regarded as one of the virus's "proofs."[61] However, as argued by Dr. Mark Bailey—who represents the No Virus position—the experiments lacked valid control comparisons, specifically with regard to environmental conditions. So, the damage that the plants underwent could have been explained by the environment rather than an alleged invisible virus. Thus, Dr. Bailey remarks that the experiments were "unscientific and inconclusive." Ivanovsky even commented, "This disease finds favourable conditions of existence only in coastal regions. Such a conclusion fully agrees with the [experiment's] observations concerning the influence of moisture on the development of the disease. Mosaic disease appears to be unique to humid and warm climates." In response, Dr. Bailey writes: "As germ theory was developing into the predominant disease-causation ideology at that time, rather than concluding that the Mosaic Disease was caused by environmental conditions, Ivanovsky concluded he had discovered an invisible virus."[62]

Even if one were to disregard the study's faulty design, the study, at best, could only develop a conclusion based on indirect evidence—since no virus was actually seen.[63] This is a far cry from the declaration that the Tobacco Mosaic Virus was the first virus to be discovered (as Wikipedia reports[64]).

In 1911, Peyton Rous at the Rockefeller Institute in New York reportedly discovered a virus—a "transmissible agent"—that causes tumors in chickens (later named the Rous sarcoma virus), for which he won a Nobel Prize in 1966. Dr. Bailey provides a critique, however. He notes that a virus was not isolated, that the experiment's controls were improper, and that the mechanism of causing disease in the experiment was unlike anything that would occur in nature. And since the electron microscope hadn't been invented yet, no virus was seen. As Dr. Bailey puts it:

> A review of [Rous's] paper, "A Sarcoma of the Fowl," reveals that he did not claim to isolate anything, let alone anything that met the definition of a virus. His methodology involved grinding up chicken tumour material, filtering it, and injecting it directly into other chickens with the observation that some of them would also develop tumours. He reported that the "control" experiments consisted of injecting unfiltered tumour material into chickens which tended to result in much larger tumours. Rous postulated the presence of a causative ultramicroscopic organism but conceded that "an agency of another sort is not out of the question."

> **Indeed, the experiment failed to provide any evidence of an infectious and replicating particle [that is, a virus]. It simply showed that diseased tissue introduced by an unnatural and invasive route into another animal could cause it to exhibit a similar disease process.**[65] [emphasis added]

The "Gold Standard" Method of Virus Isolation

In June of 1954, Thomas Peebles and Nobel laureate John Franklin Enders published a paper on a measles-virus experiment that became the gold-standard method for isolating viruses more broadly. It is the general method used in modern virology, known as the *cell-culture* method.

As virologist Dr. Stefan Lanka notes, the chronology of events is critical to understand: Dr. Enders won a Nobel Prize in December of 1954 for his work on polio that he had done in prior years. His credibility thus bolstered the status of his June 1954 paper on the measles virus, at a time when there wasn't a strong model of virology. Dr. Lanka explains the consequence: "This paper became a scientific fact which was never, ever questioned."[66] [emphasis added]

What follows is a layman's version of the study's methodology. The specific substances used can vary in modern virology, but they are similar to what Drs. Enders and Peebles used in 1954. They employed the following steps:

1. They took fluids from patients clinically diagnosed with measles, such as throat swabs.[67]
2. They mixed those fluids with a "soup" of substances, including antibiotics, bovine amniotic fluid, horse serum, beef embryo extract, milk, phenol red, soybean trypsin inhibitor, and also human and monkey kidney cells.
3. They found that some of the cells broke down once the samples from measles patients were added to the soup

(this cellular breakdown is known in virology as the *cytopathic effect*).

The conclusion was: the experiment demonstrated that a virus was in samples taken from measles patients because the samples caused cells in the soup to break down.

Certainly that's one possibility to consider, but it's not the only one—if we want to be truly scientific about this. **Here is where to really pay attention. The next few ideas are central to the No Virus position.**

How do we know that a virus was *in* the fluids from sick patients in the first place? Lots of cellular material is found in swabs from sick humans. Why wasn't the "isolated virus"—separated from all other cellular material—added to the cell culture? What if other cellular material from the throat swabs caused the cells in the soup to break down—not an alleged virus? Also, just because the patients were sick, how do we know they had a virus in the first place? They could have been sick from a host of other things.

Furthermore, what if the cell-culture-soup process itself impacts the cells, which would mean that the alleged virus was *irrelevant* in the breakdown of cells? As virologist Dr. Lanka notes, the experimenters were "killing those cells, intoxifying [*sic*] them with cytotoxic antibiotics, starving them to death, reducing the nutrition, and of course, adding material proteins which are in decay, and everything which is in decay is toxic and disturbs the cell cultures in the test tube [soup]. [Yet] when those cells are dying in the test tube, [the experimenters equate] it with the presence of the virus…and call it an 'isolate.'" **In other words, the conditions of the experiment could have caused the cells to break down—not a virus.**

Dr. Lanka also notes that the historical context needs to be considered here: the experimenters concluded that a virus was there because they were extrapolating prior discoveries about bacteria and bacteriophages. Dr. Enders was, in fact, well versed in bacteriology. So there was a presumption that alleged viruses were doing the same thing that had been observed elsewhere in the field of bacteriology. Thus, according to Dr. Lanka, the results of the 1954 experiment were biased: they were interpreted as demonstrations of the presence of a virus even though the experiment hadn't truly isolated a virus. It was just an inference.[68]

Moreover, the conclusion that a virus definitively caused cellular breakdown in the experiment is illogical. It suffers from a specific logical fallacy known as "affirming the consequent," which is summarized as:

> If P, then Q.
>
> Q, therefore P.

To put this in terminology relevant to the Enders/Peebles experiment (and to virology studies more broadly, since they employ the same basic methods):

> If there is a disease-causing virus in a sample, then it causes cells to break down.
>
> We observed that cells broke down in the experiment; therefore, there was a virus.

The logic here is defective—because alleged viruses aren't the only things that can cause cells to break down.[69] And yet this glaring error is often overlooked.

Dr. Cowan further elaborates on the problems with this gold-standard methodology as it relates to the creation of "live viral" vaccines:

> An important-to-understand corollary of [Enders's and Peebles's] precedent-setting "discoveries"—and something that almost no physician or layperson realizes—is that every "live viral vaccine" basically is nothing more than a partly purified (minimally filtered) cell-culture [soup] mixture....
>
> [In a 1957 article by Enders, he] reiterated the central dilemma: How can we know the origin of the particles that he chose to call the human measles virus? In this particular quote, he referred to the problem in the

> context of vaccines: "There is a potential risk in employing cultures of primate cells for the production of vaccines composed of attenuated virus, since the presence of other agents possibly latent in primate tissues cannot be definitively excluded by any known means."[70]

This is an important acknowledgment: there might be "agents" in the fluids other than the "virus." That is not the same as isolating *just* the "virus."

It's also worth noting that Drs. Enders and Peebles made an important admission in their paper: "Additional observations... will be required before it can be confidently asserted that [the cells in the cell-culture soup] are specifically attacked by these viruses."[71] So they weren't certain that the cell breakdown occurred *because of the alleged virus*. **The researchers also stated: "It must be borne in mind that cytopathic effects [that is, the breakdown of cells in the experiment] which superficially resemble those resulting from infection by the measles agents may possibly be induced by other viral agents present in the monkey kidney tissue...or by unknown factors."**[72] [emphasis added]

Therefore, it's clear that the authors understood that their experimental design did not *prove* that an alleged virus—which they never isolated—was responsible for the effects they found. Other factors would need to be tested in order to arrive at such a conclusion with confidence. The No Virus critique is thus that the gold-standard experiment used in modern virology does not prove the existence of a virus. And if the existence of a virus hasn't been proven, it certainly can't be proven that a non-existent thing is an intracellular parasite that causes disease in its host.

The 1954 study also lacked proper controls. Dr. Mark Bailey elaborates: "Enders and Peebles needed to identify an independent variable (the alleged virus particle) that was shown to be the cause of the cell breakdown. Their methodology was clearly insufficient in this regard and thus uncontrolled. Additionally, even if they succeeded, they would still need to establish that such particles were the cause of measles through further clinical experiments rather than just laboratory procedures."[73] Dr. Bailey adds: "Ideally, several...experiments should have been done: some with no human-derived samples added, some with human-derived samples from well [as opposed to sick] subjects, and some with human-derived samples from unwell subjects, but said not to have measles clinically or some other alleged 'viral' condition."[74]

Because modern virology studies are modeled from the foundational 1954 paper, they also lack proper controls. Dr. Bailey has evaluated countless experiments with this in mind, and he notes the following: "In many virology publications, a control or 'mock-infected' experiment is mentioned, but the details of such experiments are conspicuous by their absence."[75] Dr. Andrew Kaufman similarly reports that when he has reached out to scientists asking for details about their "mock infections," he's been unable to get straight answers from them.[76] It's not unreasonable to ask for such details, either. As Dr. Kaufman notes, *Nature*'s guidelines for the submission of scientific papers explicitly asks scientists to "include descriptions of standard protocols and experimental procedures" and "describe the experimental protocol in detail, referring to amounts of reagents in parentheses, when possible."[77]

Problems with Artificial Environments and Electron Microscopes

There's an even more fundamental issue with this gold-standard method. It has a hidden presupposition that often goes unacknowledged, and it applies not just to virology but to all sorts of biology experiments. **The studies assume that what's happening in a laboratory, test-tube environment—outside of human bodies and with very specific substances—is a close-enough proxy for what happens inside of human bodies.** But how can we be certain that what's happening to a limited number of cells in a soup represents what happens in a living, multifaceted human body that has many other complex processes occurring at once? And, moreover, should global health policies be determined on the basis of what happens in contrived, artificial, test-tube environments?[78]

These very issues lead to questions about the images seen via electron microscopes. How can we know that the pictures taken of things happening outside the body are reflective of what goes on inside the body?

The images are also static. That's problematic for identifying viruses, because they're supposed to be intracellular parasites that enter into host cells. A static image doesn't show the movement of something that performs all of the actions embedded within the modern definition of a virus.[79] Dr. Samantha Bailey elaborates on this issue:

> When the virus theory was taught to me in medical school, I believed it because I thought that sound scientific experiments must have been completed to back the theory. It wasn't until later…I investigated the literature myself and found major problems due to gaps in the evidence. It became clear that much of what was being presented as "evidence" was simply information being potentially misinterpreted in order to fit the theory. Static images are something that can easily be misinterpreted, after we assign meaning to them, that may in fact be disconnected from nature and reality. And this is where the problem of electron micrographs of what are said to be viruses needs to be explored.
>
> During my training, I would read up on a disease, such as measles, and somewhere in the chapter of a book would be an image of what was said to be the measles virus. But what had been done to show that this snapshot of some particles had confirmed that they were viruses that could cause this disease? **Was the alleged criminal really the cause of disease because somebody had pointed to it with an incriminating arrow? It kind of reminds me of accusing a person outside a bank of being a bank robber just because they were there.**[80] [emphasis added]

Additionally, the process of looking at samples under an electron microscope involves tampering with the sample.[81] That means the already problematic static image of something taken outside of a living, natural environment is *also* altered. For instance, as Dr. Bailey notes, "electron micrographs are photos of stuff that has been embedded in resin and then cut up into very thin slices. Whatever is visualized in these images is dead. The particles certainly don't replicate."[82] Also, the electron beam that's used in the microscope can cause problems because of its high energy, and related temperature changes can alter the sample.[83] Similarly, in "cryo" electron microscopy, the sample is frozen.[84]

Cellular material can also be misidentified under an electron microscope. For example, a 2020 paper in *Kidney360*, titled "Appearances Can Be Deceiving—Viral-like Inclusions in COVID-19 Negative Renal Biopsies by Electron Microscopy," warns about possible misinterpretations of electron microscopy images. Similarly, in an April 2021 article in *Emerging Infectious Diseases* on the CDC's website, titled "Difficulties in Differentiating Coronaviruses from Subcellular Structures in Human Tissues by Electron Microscopy," the authors admit to problems with electron microscopy images of SARS-CoV-2. They state: "Efforts to combat...COVID-19...have placed a renewed focus on the use of transmission electron microscopy for identifying coronavirus in tissues. In attempts to attribute pathology of COVID-19 patients directly to tissue damage caused by SARS-CoV-2, **investigators have inaccurately reported subcellular structures, including coated vesicles, multivesicular bodies, and vesiculating rough endoplasmic reticulum, as coronavirus particles.**"[85] [emphasis added]

Dr. Bailey mentions an important assertion embedded in that statement: "[The authors] are saying that to identify a virus, you need to know exactly what to look for in a structural sense. That would be a reasonable statement if they had already established that they knew exactly what a virus looks like. But how do these experts know what a virus looks like?"[86]

The study references a 1967 study in which the researchers allegedly isolated a coronavirus and took pictures, which now serves as a standard template for identifying future coronaviruses. The research was done at the Common Cold Unit that existed for nearly four decades after World War II.[87] But as Dr. Bailey notes, that 1967 study was looking at photographs of particles within a *mixture of cell-culture soups rather than isolated viruses.* The experimenters declared that certain particles seen under their electron microscope were viruses because they looked like *another* "virus" seen elsewhere, called "avian infectious bronchitis virus." And that particle type, as Dr. Bailey explains, "has never been properly isolated either." The experimenters also never demonstrated that the particles under the microscope were parasitic in nature—as viruses are said to be. She thus describes the images as "cellular vesicles of unknown significance" rather than "viruses." All future researchers looking into coronaviruses are "building on an unestablished premise" (in Dr. Bailey's words). She humorously refers to the images as UVOs (unidentified viral objects).[88]

Furthermore, it's important for electron micrographs to be taken of control groups as well. The No Virus contention is that control images aren't taken. In fact, since the independent variable (the hypothesized virus) hasn't been isolated, a proper control is an impossibility.[89] Therefore, the researchers can't know if what they're seeing under a microscope would show up anyway—even if an alleged virus hadn't been added.[90]

The No Virus camp is thus unconvinced by virology studies that show pictures of things claimed to be viruses—if the scientific method isn't properly followed. **Dr. Lanka summarizes the situation well: "Virologists never, ever saw a virus inside the living being or inside its liquids....Everybody can check it easily on every single photograph that should show a virus—that it's from a cell culture [soup]. But never from the blood, never from the saliva, never from the semen, never from another liquid of the body. Never from a lymph node. Never from the inside. Not from a human, not from an animal, not from a plant. This is astonishing....They never managed to get a virus photographed inside a human being."**[91] (Note: When interviewing Dr. Lanka, Dr. Thomas Cowan mentioned that he's looked for scientific papers describing the morphology of a virus from a living, diseased person. He says there are a few papers that *claim* to have done so, but after reading the details, the scientists say the things they find have very *different* morphologies—meaning they look different. Therefore, it's unlikely that they are actually all the same virus. So the experimenters are likely seeing other cellular material that's being mistakenly called a "virus."[92]) [emphasis added]

Sequencing Genomes

The No Virus position here is ultimately very simple. It was alluded to previously but warrants another mention because this is such a hot topic. In order to generate a genetic sequence of something, first that thing needs to be isolated; then its genetic sequence can be determined. Without first isolating *just the virus*, how can it be known that the genetic material that's being analyzed comes from the virus specifically? In the absence of pure virus isolation, genetic material taken from samples could be from other debris. This makes CRISPR's alleged "virus" detection techniques inherently problematic—and the same goes for any other genetic testing technology. (Note: On a related topic, *any* material alleged to "come from a virus" such as "spike proteins" can't be known to come from a virus if the virus hasn't been isolated first. Cellular material might have origins that have nothing to do with a virus.[93])

Consider Dr. Mark Bailey's criticism of the original genetic sequencing of SARS-CoV-2. He explains that the team of scientists "assembled an *in silico* 'genome' from **genetic fragments of unknown provenance**, found in the crude lung washings of a single 'case' [of SARS-CoV-2]."[94] *In silico* refers to a computational model of a hypothesized genome; that is, the genome doesn't exist in its entirety in the experiment at all.[95] As Dr. Kaufman notes, an *in silico* genome is an "artificial version of something that doesn't exist. It is a model or a simulation." In essence, it's man-made.[96] [emphasis added]

And yet, the original alleged genetic sequencing of SARS-CoV-2 was not positioned to the public with such caveats. Dr. Bailey adds: "A virus is claimed to be a tiny replication-competent obligate intracellular parasite.…It is an infectious particle that *causes* disease in a host. All [the authors of the SARS-CoV-2 genetic sequencing paper] had was a 41-year old man with pneumonia and a software-assembled model 'genome' made from sequences of unestablished origin found in the man's lung washings."[97] [emphasis added]

Additionally, Dr. Bailey criticizes the lack of controls used. Controls would entail, for example, running the sequencing process on a variety of samples, including those without the alleged virus.[98]

Furthermore, from the No Virus perspective, alleged "variants" of viruses are just combinations of genetic fragments that are patched together in a computer to create a slightly different overall result. Various "template" genomes are established, so scientists can look for something specific; and if they find a match, they can declare that they found a variant of the virus. But the same problems persist in this process: without an isolated virus, scientists cannot be certain of the genetic material's origin.

Put another way by Dr. Kaufman, the identification of alleged "variants" is simply an inability to find an exact match of previously patched-together genomes. But instead of interpreting them as failures to reproduce results, researchers just call them "variants."[99]

For further information on the No Virus position regarding genetic sequencing—a highly technical matter—see Dr. Bailey's "A Farewell to Virology."[100]

"Antiviral" Drugs

Without first isolating a virus, inventing a drug that helps the body fight the unidentified virus is an impossibility. Yet antiviral drugs exist. What does the No Virus group think this class of drugs is doing?

In response to a question along these lines posed by podcast host Tom Woods in February 2023, Dr. Bailey replied: "None of [these antivirals] act against viruses....[Mainstream virologists allege] that [a viral] particle goes inside a host cell, such as a human cell, and uses the cell's equipment to make more copies of itself. So essentially an 'antiviral' [drug] just has to interfere with some process within the host cell. **So they're not antivirals. They're just antimetabolic agents basically....Maybe the closest analogy would be chemotherapy. It's not attacking the cancer cell, per se. It's an antimetabolite. It's stopping processes from happening [and] slowing them down within the cell."**[101] [emphasis added]

Dr. Bailey has further noted that antiviral drugs are claimed to prevent the "virus" from replicating. Researchers determine this by looking at particular nucleic acid (DNA or RNA) levels in a test-tube environment and find that there is less produced when the antiviral is added. That is, the "viral load" is diminished.

However, as just discussed, the *origin* of such genetic sequences cannot be declared as viral without isolating a virus *first*. Dr. Bailey remarks, "The genetic sequences in such experiments could be produced endogenously (from within the cell) **which does not require the existence of the alleged virus**. An example concerning SARS-CoV-2 was when researchers in Australia reported they were 'able to effect ~5000-fold reduction in virus' with the drug Ivermectin. In reality, they were only measuring cell-culture RNA levels with the unfounded claim that the RNA was known to come from a virus."[102]

The No Virus camp thus contends that the effects and mechanisms of "antiviral" drugs are misinterpreted by modern researchers.

Factors Allegedly Preventing Virus Isolation

The "ask" of the No Virus camp seems pretty simple: they want scientists to follow the scientific method so that it can be determined whether viruses, as currently defined, exist and cause disease. They want an isolated virus—that is, an independent variable—and they want proper controls. However, the status quo defends its current methods. Dr. Thomas Cowan describes a common experience among No Virus proponents:

> When I ask doctors or virologists why they don't carry out [a] simple, clear, logical, rational proof to demonstrate

> the existence of a new virus and show it causes disease, I hear one of two answers. The first is that not enough of the virus is present in any bodily fluid of any sick person to find it in this way. [For instance, Dr. Kaufman] even asked scientists whether they would see the virus if the bronchial fluid from 10,000 people with "COVID" were pooled, but the response is the same: "There is not enough virus to find." This, of course, begs the question: On what theory are we then claiming the virus is making people sick? To this, there is no answer.[103]

Put another way, if there isn't "enough virus" for it to be studied, then what is the mechanism by which it is so contagious, and in some cases, deadly? And furthermore, how do they know that there isn't enough of the virus…if they're admitting that they haven't isolated it in the first place?

In fact, the argument that Dr. Cowan references is the same one that Dr. Luc Montagnier made when he acknowledged "we did not purify" (in his 1983 HIV work). Dr. Montagnier elaborated in an interview in 1997: "There was so little production of the virus [that] it was impossible to see what might be in a concentrate of the virus from the gradient ['pure virus']. There was not enough virus to do that."[104]

Dr. Cowan continues: "The second answer I have heard [in defense of virology's typical methods] is that viruses are intracellular 'parasites'—so, of course, we can't find them outside the cells. When asked how the virus passes from one person to another, as we are told it does, virologists reply, 'It buds out of the cell, goes into a droplet and travels to the next person.' In other words, the virus is transmitted when it is outside of the cell. I can only wonder why virologists can't find it during this transmission step since they clearly think it is outside the cell."[105]

Another defense of virology's methods is that the technology doesn't exist to isolate particles as small as viruses. However, Dr. Kaufman argues that exosomes and bacteriophages, which are similarly sized, *have* been isolated. He points to representative studies to back up his claim.[106] Dr. Stefan Lanka adds, "These [bacteriophages] could be photographed, isolated as whole particles, and all their components could be biochemically determined and characterized. This is real, and cannot be contested....This, however, has never happened with alleged viruses of humans, animals, and plants because these do not exist."[107]

Finally, the HART organization—a group of distinguished doctors, scientists, and other academics in the United Kingdom—published a critique of the No Virus position in an October 2023 article. **They explicitly acknowledge that "there has never been a pure isolate of SARS-CoV-2 virus." Incredibly, they then remark: "This could be because no-one [*sic*] has tried hard enough to carry out this work."** Their article also refers to "the virus *model*." This is an admission that, even from a mainstream perspective, the notion of a contagious, disease-causing virus has not been firmly established. (Note: For a point-by-point rebuttal of the article's contentions, see Dr. Cowan's October 11, 2023, webinar alongside Dr. Mark Bailey.[108]) [emphasis added]

Dr. Stefan Lanka's Control Study

One might rightly ask: If the No Virus perspective is correct about something so fundamental, why don't its advocates simply conduct their own laboratory experiments to demonstrate the flaws in modern virology? Why don't they run proper controls on their own? Going forward, this would be an important strategy for the No Virus camp, *if they can obtain the funding to do so*. Scientific journals would likely be reluctant to publish such research, but the studies could still be done. It also takes brave scientists to engage in such a matter. They could be risking their careers.

There is one noteworthy instance, however. The study was conducted by Dr. Stefan Lanka in 2021 and, not surprisingly, it wasn't published in a mainstream journal. He sought to study whether cell breakdown occurs in cell-culture soups...without adding fluids from a sick person believed to be sick from a virus. In other words, he wanted to see if the various substances in cell-culture soups cause cells to break down *on their own*. This is the sort of control study that the No Virus camp had been asking for.

Dr. Cowan summarizes the results:

> [One of Dr. Lanka's trials] shows what happened when [he] used the same procedures that have been used in every modern isolation of every pathogenic virus that I have seen. This included changing the nutrient medium to "minimal nutrient medium"—meaning lowering the percentage of fetal calf serum from the usual 10% to 1%, which lowers the nutrients available for the cells to grow, thereby stressing them—and tripling the antibiotic concentration....On day five of the experiment, the characteristic [cell breakdown] occurred, "proving" the existence and pathogenicity of the virus—**except, at no point was a pathogenic virus added to the culture. This outcome can only mean that the [cell breakdown] was a result of the way the culture experiment was done and not from any virus.**[109] [emphasis added]

Dr. Lanka ran another trial just like this one, except that he added yeast RNA—rather than fluids from a person sick from an alleged virus—to the cell-culture soup. Again, the cells in the soup broke down.[110]

Thus, these trials demonstrate that cellular breakdown in classic virology experiments *can occur without a virus*. The implication—if extended beyond this experiment—is that the gold-standard virology experiments aren't proving the existence of a disease-causing virus. In other words, the effect that scientists typically see could be an artifact of the way the experiment is set up.

***Many* more similar experiments and independent replications are needed, but Dr. Lanka's results lend initial support to the No Virus camp's position.** Also, No Virus proponents have found some examples in virology papers suggesting that the procedure itself can cause cells to break down—which supports Dr. Lanka's findings.[111]

Challenges to Virology Prevail in German Courts

For those who accept Dr. Lanka's results, they are powerful and certainly challenge the core of virology. But No Virus advocates also find hope in court victories in Germany—two instances in particular. The first relates to a 2011 challenge issued by Dr. Lanka: he offered 100,000 euros to anyone who could show scientific evidence that the measles virus exists. He did this because he was concerned about a growing momentum to mandate the measles vaccine for children in Germany. In 2015, physician David Bardens sued Dr. Lanka for 100,000 euros because he submitted six papers which, in his mind, proved the existence of the measles virus. Dr. Samantha Bailey analyzed the six papers and gave a summary as to why they don't show virus isolation:[112]

1. The 1954 Enders and Peebles study (the problems with its cell-culture-soup design have already been discussed).[113]

2. A 1958 cell-culture experiment similar to the Enders and Peebles study, which suffered from the same problems.[114]

3. A 1969 paper showing many pictures of alleged viruses but lacked evidence that the photographs were of viruses. The particles also weren't established to be infectious or disease-causing.[115]

4. A 1984 paper in which the authors showed purified particles that they claimed to be measles viruses, but lacked evidence that they were in fact measles viruses that cause disease.[116]

5. A 1995 consensus review paper in which the authors claimed to describe the measles virus genome.[117] As Dr. Bailey puts it: "This [genome] was based on detecting genetic fragments in test tubes and assembling them into a hypothetical model. It was not established that the computer-generated sequence exists in nature."

6. A 2007 paper describing a classic cell-culture experiment with monkey kidney cells, which ran no controls and had the same methodological problems that all virology studies do.[118]

A lower court in Germany—which did not rely on expert-witness testimony—ordered Dr. Lanka to pay Dr. Bardens, and the media jumped on the story. **What the media talks about much less is the fact that Dr. Lanka appealed the case and won in 2016.** Dr. Bardens then appealed to the highest court in Germany, and his appeal was dismissed.[119] So Dr. Lanka ultimately won.

Skeptics claim that Dr. Lanka only won because of a technicality or a semantic formulation. However, during the proceedings, Andreas Podbielski—a professor in the department of medical microbiology and virology in Rostock—admitted that none of the six papers that Dr. Bardens submitted had been done with proper controls.[120] As Dr. Samantha Bailey summarizes the situation: **"The best six papers in the entire measles 'virus' literature didn't follow the scientific method."[121]** [emphasis added]

The second victory in the German court system came in April 2023 at the hands of engineer Marvin Haberland. He wanted to challenge COVID-19 lockdown measures, so he intentionally violated a local mask mandate and was fined, which enabled him to present a case in court.

Germany's COVID-19 policies were dependent on the Law for the Prevention and Control of Infectious Diseases in Humans. The first paragraph of the law suggested that institutions needed to abide by science—meaning they needed to follow the scientific method. Haberland comments that he heard Dr. Lanka—who is one of his "heroes"—once suggest that if a person receives a fine, the strategy should be to point to the first paragraph of the law and argue that it's not fulfilled because virology does not follow the scientific method. And if paragraph one is not fulfilled, then the rest of the law should become irrelevant.

Haberland decided to use this exact argument in his case. He even asked virologists around the world about their "control"

studies. He reports: "None of them carried out the controls, and they even admit that....They really admit that they do not do any scientific controls....For the first step [of virus isolation experiments], which is the [cell breakdown step] they will sometimes *say* they do [controls], but when they are asked to provide documentation or evidence on how they did it, they also cannot do it."[122] He adds, "We have hundreds of letters from virologists all over the world confirming they have not done the control experiments—specifically in the genome sequencing—nobody has done them." [emphasis added]

In 2023, the judge assigned to Haberland's case decided to close the case—which was an effective concession and a victory for Haberland. Four others replicated Haberland's template, and the same thing happened: the court closed the cases. As Haberland puts it: "If the court had any possible chance to win, they would use the [opportunity] to try to somehow make a precedent and show everyone, 'Look, these [No Virus] people are stupid. They have no chance, and virology is actually a [legitimate] thing.' But they didn't make this case." In other words, Haberland feels that the judge closed his case "to avoid any further damage to virology." He also speculates that the judge could have put himself in danger if he had allowed virology's problems to be exposed so publicly.[123]

Freedom of Information Challenges

Governments around the world have also admitted to virology's failure to physically isolate viruses. The admissions have come through "freedom of information" (FOI) submissions led by biostatistician Christine Massey of Canada. FOI requests allow everyday citizens in many countries to obtain access to records that aren't already in the public domain. In June 2023, Massey summarized the state of the FOI process:

> Myself and people around the world have taken advantage of this process to seek records that would be necessary in order for anyone to show the existence of the alleged COVID-19 virus (SARS-CoV-2). And if somebody actually wanted to conduct science and show

> that there is a virus that is infecting people, they would need to actually find it in order to [genetically] sequence and characterize a particle and study it. With controlled experiments...you would actually have to have a sample of this alleged virus to work with. And if nobody has a sample of the alleged virus, then nobody can have conducted any science. And so this is what the majority of these FOI requests were focused on. We were asking for any records of anyone in the world ever finding this alleged virus in the bodily fluid or tissue or excrement of any people anywhere on Earth by anyone, ever.
>
> **And to date, we have responses from 216 different institutions in forty different countries, and so far no one has been able to provide us with even one record. They can't provide us with even one record, and they can't cite any record. So they've all admitted that they don't have a sample of the alleged virus, and they don't even know of anyone else who did obtain a sample of this alleged virus.**[124] [emphasis added]

For example, the first record obtained was from the CDC (with letterhead from the US Department of Health and Human Services [HHS]) on November 2, 2020, in response to a FOI request. The request asked for:

> All records in the possession, custody, or control of the Centers for Disease Control (CDC) describing the isolation of the SARS-COV-2 virus, directly from a sample from a diseased patient, where the sample was not first combined with any other source of genetic material (i.e., monkey kidney cells aka vero cells; lung cells from a lung cancer patient).
>
> Please note that I am using "isolation" in the everyday sense of the word: the act of separating a thing(s) from everything else. I am not requesting records where "isolation of SARS-COV-2" refers instead to: the culturing of something; or the performance of an amplification test (i.e., a PCR test); or the sequencing of something.

> Please note that my request is not limited to records that were authored by the CDC or that pertain to work done by the CDC. My request includes any sort of record, for example (but not limited to) any published peer-reviewed study that the CDC has downloaded or printed.
>
> If any such records match the above description of requested records and are currently available to the public elsewhere, please provide enough information about each record so that I may identify and access each record with certainty (i.e., title, author[s], date, journal, where the public may access it).[125]

The response from the CDC, via the HHS, was: "A search of our records failed to reveal any documents pertaining to your request."[126] [emphasis added]

Massey notes that in all of the responses starting from March 1, 2021, the CDC "stopped admitting flat out that they didn't have any records. They started giving more convoluted responses to make it sound like they do have science when they actually don't. And [they direct] us to irrelevant studies."

A March 1, 2021, response from the CDC stated: "The definition of 'isolation' provided in the request is outside of what is possible in virology."[127] So the CDC is saying that isolating an independent variable in a scientific experiment, which is necessary in order to do science, is not possible. It's an explicit admission, as the No Virus group sees it, that virology is not practicing science. [emphasis added]

In another request, Massey's team asked for details about control methods used in virus isolation studies and the whole genome sequencing of SARS-CoV-2. The UK Health Agency responded on March 25, 2022, by citing a "national security" exemption, arguing that releasing details would "directly contravene an explicit request from the World Health Organization."[128]

Massey decided to expand the search beyond SARS-CoV-2, asking government agencies to point her to evidence for the isolation of *any* alleged virus from any diseased person. In a December 20, 2021, response from the Public Health Agency of Canada, the answer was: "Your request resulted in a 'No Records Exist,' because of the way that you have formulated your request. The isolation of a virus cannot be completed without the use of another medium....The gold standard assay used to determine the presence of intact virus in patient samples is virus isolation in cell culture."[129] However, as discussed earlier, the No Virus argument contends that the so-called gold-standard, cell-culture-soup method is highly problematic. And this is the point that the No Virus camp makes: the field of virology is presupposing that the gold-standard method dating back to 1954 is valid, when apparently few scientists have gone back to question the foundation on which the entire field is based.

Massey has also started to request evidence for the isolation of other viruses specifically. She's received responses from various agencies around the world, and so far they have been unable to provide records for the following "viruses": adenovirus, Ebolavirus, Epstein-Barr, hepatitis B and C, herpes, HIV, HPV, H1N1 (swine flu), H5N1 (avian flu), lentivirus, Marburg virus, measles, MERS, monkeypox, rabies, RSV, SARS (or any other common-cold-associated coronaviruses), smallpox, West Nile, XMRV, and Zika.[130]

These are startling results.

Settling the Virus Debate

Dr. Mark Bailey sums up the No Virus position well: "One of the pivotal issues with virology was that it invented itself as a field before establishing if viruses actually existed. It has been trying to justify itself since its inception."[131]

The fundamental problems discussed in this chapter thus give reason to doubt a key element of germ-focused allopathic medicine. There isn't much of a middle ground here: either you believe there are deadly viruses that can be transmitted from person to person—and live with the appropriate precautions—or you don't. From a public-health-policy perspective, the differences are massive. Lockdowns, mask regulations, vaccine mandates, business shutdowns, surveillance, and all of the measures we've experienced during the COVID-19 era would make no sense if the deadly virus justifying the measures didn't exist in the way that we've been told. Furthermore, without an "invisible enemy," any future pandemics—and associated tyrannical measures—wouldn't be possible. So this is far more than an intellectual exercise.

A proposed method to resolve the matter was outlined by twenty doctors, scientists, and researchers in July of 2022—all of whom signed a document titled "Settling the Virus Debate."[132] It lays out the precise scientific protocols that multiple virology labs around the world could conduct. As of the time of this writing, more than a year after the document's publication, there haven't been any takers. (Note: Dr. Stefan Lanka did *not* include his name as a signatory because he feels that virology has already been refuted and there isn't a need to offer virology any more challenges.[133])

An overarching hurdle for the No Virus position is that a negative can't be proven. It's not possible to prove that something doesn't exist. But, at the same time, it also can't be proven that a "flying spaghetti monster" doesn't exist.[134] There's always the possibility: "Maybe we just haven't found it yet."

CHAPTER 3

HOW TO DEMONSTRATE THAT A GERM CAUSES DISEASE

Given what's been discussed so far—a troubled medical system in the introduction, HIV/AIDS anomalies in chapter 1, and questions about virology in chapter 2—taking another look at a variety of allegedly infectious diseases seems warranted.

But a prerequisite to that is understanding which methodology should be used in order to properly determine that germs *cause* disease—in a logical and scientific manner. That's the subject of this chapter, whereas the next chapter examines specific diseases, one by one.

Koch's Postulates

The standard method for showing that germs cause disease comes from the work of the late-19th-century researcher Dr. Robert Koch. Various versions of his "postulates" are often presented, but they share the same logic. They are far more thorough than merely saying, "People got sick; therefore, it must be the case that a microscopic bacteria or virus caused the sickness."

In fact, in 2003, the WHO stated that "conclusive identification of a causative [agent] must meet all criteria of the so-called

Koch's postulate [*sic*]." Dr. Mark Bailey points out in his paper "A Farewell to Virology" (2022) that the WHO's article has since been removed from its website but can be accessed using the internet archive.[1] [emphasis added]

What follows is a simplified version of "Koch's postulates" (adapted from a synopsis provided by Dr. Samantha Bailey):[2]

1. The microorganism must be found in the ill but not the healthy.
2. The microorganism must be isolated from a diseased organism and grown in pure culture.
3. The microorganism must produce the same disease in another host.
4. The microorganism must be re-isolated from that new host.

Rethinking Bacteria

Dr. Koch won a Nobel Prize in 1905 for his work on the alleged bacterial infection tuberculosis (TB). Some who have examined the details of his methods challenge the claim that he truly demonstrated, in an appropriately scientific manner, that the bacterium is the cause of disease.[3] But there's a problem that is even more fundamental than his techniques. The WHO states: "About 5–10% of people infected with TB will eventually get symptoms and develop TB disease."[4] Koch's first postulate entails that in order for a microorganism to be established as the causative agent of disease—meaning that it, and not some other factor, results in disease—*only* sick people should have the microorganism. **If healthy people also have the microorganism in their bodies, then there must be some other factor that is causing illness in the small percentage that do get sick.**

Furthermore, one of Dr. Bailey's colleagues submitted requests to various health organizations in New Zealand, asking for studies and reports that use purified bacteria to prove causation of the TB disease. He specified that he did not want studies that failed to fulfill Koch's postulates or didn't use valid controls. Dr. Bailey reports on the "funniest" response, which came from the New Zealand Ministry of Health. It didn't have the information requested and didn't believe that any other organization would have the information either. Instead, the Ministry of Health issued a reminder that Dr. Koch won a Nobel Prize for demonstrating that a tuberculosis bacterium causes TB (as if his credentials acted as a sufficient substitute for scientific evidence—which it didn't).[5]

Ironically, the failure to meet Koch's postulates is often excused by calling them "out of date"—this is in spite of the WHO's 2003 comment to the contrary, as just mentioned.[6] However, the postulates are entirely logical. They simply represent a problem for allopathic medicine: when scientists fail to meet the postulates faithfully, it puts into question germ-based contagion.

Alternatively, perhaps the failure to meet Koch's postulates reflects a fundamental misunderstanding about the nature and role of bacteria. These microorganisms appear, in great abundance, in healthy people. For instance, *E. coli* bacteria live in the intestines of healthy people,[7] and *Staphylococcus* bacteria live on healthy people's skin.[8] Typically, *E. coli* and staph are associated with scary "infections." But since the bacteria live in healthy people, Koch's first postulate is not fulfilled—the bacteria are not the cause of disease.

An emerging perspective in "alternative" health circles is that bacteria cannot be disease-causing agents in the way they've been made out to be. On the contrary, bacteria exist within us symbiotically as a "cleanup crew." In nature, bacteria are scavengers that decompose decaying material (the technical term is that they are *saprophytic*).[9] In fact, fungi and parasites could be looked at similarly: they are uniquely capable of cleaning things up—and perhaps that's why they exist in humans. It's akin to the way in which maggots only eat dead tissue: they appear on carcasses, but they weren't the killers.

So, under this perspective, if bacteria are found at the scene, that indicates there's an underlying issue or toxicity that they're assisting with.[10] Recall that firefighters appearing at the scene of a fire doesn't imply that firefighters *caused* the fire. The same might be true with bacteria, fungi, and parasites. They get blamed for something they didn't do.

Bacteria *can* emit toxins, however (such as endotoxins, cholera toxin, and botulinum toxin).[11] Those toxins can be viewed as waste products of bacteria rather than a venomous defense mechanism (as pointed out by Dr. Andrew Kaufman).[12] But even if bacterial toxins incidentally cause damage to their surroundings, that still doesn't suggest that bacteria fundamentally *cause* disease on their own. From the alternative view discussed here, bacteria only show up in great quantities to "put out fires" within the body. If those fires hadn't been there, the bacteria (and their toxic waste products) wouldn't have been such a big concern in the first place.

Dr. Samantha Bailey elaborates on this notion, specifically regarding TB:

> The truth of the matter is that the [bacteria responsible for TB] are everywhere. We inhale and ingest the bacteria all the time. But according to germ theory, by some miracle, most of us never get the condition known as TB. People with TB don't "catch" the disease, as epidemiological studies fallaciously conclude.
>
> The areas where the disease is rampant are afflicted by common factors. If an individual is [in an otherwise] poor condition, then the bacteria that are already present in the lungs in small numbers will start to proliferate. **They have no capacity to launch an attack against healthy tissue and are the cleanup crew for compromised and dirty tissue. That's why TB is seen in IV drug users, homeless people, third-world counties, individuals with cancer, and those taking drugs known as immunosuppressants. These are all toxic situations, and the solution is not isolating them or filling them up with more pharmaceuticals....The**

> **remedy is reversing the underlying toxicities and addressing their malnourishment.**[13] [emphasis added]

Furthermore, Christine Massey and her colleagues (mentioned in the previous chapter) have begun to aggregate Freedom of Information requests sent to health agencies that ask for evidence of disease caused by various bacteria. So far, the agencies have been unable to provide evidence that bacteria *cause* disease.[14] (Note: The implication is *not* that people don't need to wash their hands. Hands can still become dirty with harmful contaminants. This topic is covered in further detail in Dr. Bailey's video titled *5 Spectacular Fails from Germ Theory*.[15]) [emphasis added]

These ideas challenge allopathic thinking, and there's often a desire to defend the status quo. For instance, the story of John Snow, MD, is sometimes invoked as proof of bacterial contagion: he was able to stop a cholera outbreak in London in 1854 by removing the handle of a water pump (known as the Broad Street pump). However, the belief that a bacterial infection was to blame is unwarranted, according to Dr. Bailey. She explains that the river was heavily contaminated by cesspools, formed from sewers and filth, which the London government dumped into the Thames River. In Dr. Bailey's words:

> While Snow's analysis was correct in concluding that it was contaminated water making people sick, the modern-era story that it was an infection from the bacterium *Vibrio cholerae* is not. To this day, there is no scientific evidence that the ingestion of bacteria by itself will make anyone sick. Max von Pettenkofer first demonstrated this in 1892 by swallowing a large culture of *Vibrio cholerae* provided by Robert Koch. Disappointingly for Koch, his rival did not succumb to cholera.... However, the ingestion of fecal material, decomposing biological tissue, and other toxins can certainly make people sick. So the cluster of cases in London had nothing to do with infection and everything to do with a common factor of drinking filthy, waste-containing river-Thames water.[16]

Faithfully following a methodology like Koch's postulates can avoid confusion like this. They allow scientists to logically determine whether a bacterium is the *cause* of disease. **Instead, as is often the case, people fall into the trap of jumping to conclusions based on epidemiological observations (that is, noting patterns of sickness within a population). Epidemiology alone doesn't establish the *cause* of sickness—additional scientific analyses are needed to sift through a host of possibilities.**[17]

Rivers's Postulates

Koch's postulates came about at a time when no technology existed that could see particles as small as viruses are alleged to be. So, even though the overall methodology is sound enough to be applied to viruses, it wasn't "made" for viruses. When improved technology emerged several decades later, Thomas Rivers updated the postulates for viruses. Dr. Thomas Cowan and Sally Fallon Morell provide a basic summary of what they are:[18]

1. The virus can be isolated from diseased hosts.
2. The virus can be cultivated in host cells.
3. The virus can be filtered from a medium that also contains bacteria (known as *proof of filterability*).
4. The filtered virus will produce a comparable disease when the cultivated virus is used to infect experimental animals.
5. The virus can be reisolated from the infected experimental animal.
6. A specific immune response to the virus can be detected.

Dr. Cowan and Morell comment:

> Rivers dropped Koch's first postulate....Even with Koch's first postulate missing, researchers have not been able to prove that a specific virus causes a specific disease using Rivers's postulates; one study claims that Rivers's postulates have been met for SARS, said to be a viral

> disease, but careful examination of the paper demonstrates that none of the postulates have been satisfied.
>
> **No disease attributed to bacteria or viruses has met all of Koch's postulates or all of Rivers's criteria. This is not because the postulates are incorrect or obsolete (in fact, they are entirely logical), but rather because bacteria and viruses don't cause disease, at least not in any way that we currently understand.**[19] [emphasis added]

(Note: This above extract comes from Dr. Cowan and Morell's 2020 book, *The Contagion Myth*. It was banned from Amazon. The book was renamed *The Truth About Contagion* and then was allowed to be sold on Amazon.[20])

From the perspective of the No Virus camp, it would make sense that these postulates haven't been fulfilled for viruses…*because their view is that no virus has ever been isolated.* Without an isolated virus, the later postulates are irrelevant. But researchers might claim in their papers that they did fulfill Rivers's postulates, even though they did not, because they don't acknowledge the flaws of the gold-standard virus isolation method (as discussed in chapter 2).

Furthermore, because of the lack of true virus isolation, diagnosing alleged viral illnesses is inherently problematic. It often relies on *indirect* testing methods, such as looking for the presence of "antibodies" or detecting genetic fragments with a PCR test. As we saw with HIV/AIDS, the tests were often unreliable, and the same thing has occurred during the COVID-19 era. In other instances, diagnoses are made on the basis of symptoms alone. But that subjective method doesn't prove that a particular pathogen is the *cause* of the observed symptoms. Observations, by themselves, don't prove causation.[21]

Drs. Cowan, Samantha and Mark Bailey, and others have been asking mainstream germ theorists for nearly four years to present papers that truly meet Koch's and Rivers's postulates, and they haven't seen any. **Given how ubiquitous germ theory is, one might expect there to be hundreds or thousands of papers that clearly**

demonstrate—with proper scientific methods and controls—that specific germs *cause* disease and can be passed from person to person. And yet that doesn't seem to be the case.

As Dr. Mark Bailey says, "We encourage people to send [studies allegedly proving contagion] to us. And most people have given up doing that because we've critiqued all of the major ones."[22] Dr. Samantha Bailey thus concludes, "Aerosol transmission of microbes that cause disease has never been demonstrated in the history of medical science, and it is a fairy tale to scare children and naive adults."[23]

This camp subscribes to what's known as "terrain theory"—the notion that one's "terrain" (that is, one's body and mind) is central to health, similar to the way in which healthy soil results in healthy plants. Terrain theorists focus on the terrain; germ theorists focus on the germ. Terrain theory is a threat to allopathic medicine.[24]

Dr. Mark Bailey aptly points out some important caveats within terrain theory. Terrain theory doesn't deny that microorganisms can result in bodily harm under certain circumstances. **When our own body is breaking down, germs can flourish in dangerous quantities.** Moreover, in large enough quantities *anything* can be injurious—even drinking unnatural amounts of water is unsafe. It's even possible that a biological weapon could combine a chemical with bacteria such that the chemical would damage the body's terrain and allow the bacteria to proliferate. Dr. Bailey further adds that "the ingestion of decomposing biological tissue is harmful to us: the oldest 'biological weapon' during sieges was poisoning the enemy's water supply with rotting animal corpses."[25]

Overall, however, terrain theorists flip the script on the nature and role of often-vilified microbes: they go from being the enemy to being essential helpers. The fact that they exist in nature and assist our bodies, even though we didn't "ask" them to, implies that nature is more friendly to humans than we've been led to believe. The typical "enemy," from the terrain-theorist's perspective, is ourselves: we poison ourselves through toxic chemicals in virtually everything we use, eat, and drink; our drugs are toxic; our air is often unclean; we're surrounded by electricity and wireless radiation; and we often suffer from poor diets, a lack of sleep and exercise, not enough time in nature or under natural sunlight, and patterns of toxic emotions and unprocessed trauma. All of these considerations might impact our health and can manifest as various forms of illness or even death.

These ideas are not top of mind for allopathic germ theorists; they are secondary. Additionally, the culprits under terrain theory (in addition to ourselves) are huge industries that produce toxins, radiation, and harmful drugs, whereas germ theory points the finger at invisible microbes. Germ theory keeps the attention away from those who might actually be causing damage. Thus, there is an economic incentive to make germ theory prominent in the public's psyche.

If the terrain theorists are correct, then a huge part of the allopathic model—and its approach to diagnosing and treating disease—is massively off base. In fact, there are many anomalies that support terrain theory, as I will discuss in the next chapter.

CHAPTER 4

REVISITING INFECTIOUS DISEASES

This chapter covers a wide variety of allegedly infectious diseases, presenting an alternative view from the terrain-theory perspective—one that views "diseases" as symptoms of something other than infectious germs that can pass from person to person. I broached this in chapter 1 regarding HIV/AIDS, and what follows here is a much more concise look at many other well-known illnesses.

More than anything, the goal here is to establish a pattern of critical thinking. This is often lacking today, as the public is conditioned to reflexively think that a germ must have caused disease if people get sick in the same place. The analyses also aim to resolve questions that might be arising in your minds about diseases previously assumed to be contagious. Also, this mode of critical thinking naturally puts into question whether vaccines are the "saviors" that modern culture often views them to be.

With that context in mind, the exemplary set of "infectious diseases" covered in this chapter includes polio, SARS, Spanish flu, avian flu, smallpox, chicken pox, hepatitis, rabies, and the Black Death.

The intent of this analysis is *not to present with certainty* a definitive narrative for each illness, but rather to open minds to new possibilities—in the spirit of questioning allopathic assumptions. The unfortunate reality is that modern medicine often doesn't know the full story as to why and how illness arises, because humanity's understanding of biology and the nature of reality is in its infancy.[1]

Furthermore, since the allopathic model dominates modern medicine, the majority of research goes toward allopathic hypotheses. The flip side of this dynamic is that other viewpoints garner less support—and funding—which means that many of them remain hypothetical. Therefore, mainstream skeptics can fall back on the criticism that "these alternative explanations lack sufficient evidence"...because most of the research dollars are being directed toward germ theory. Allopathic medicine thus perpetuates itself. A first step toward breaking the cycle is to question assumptions and formulate new hypotheses that need to be tested.

Given how much sickness persists in modern society, such a radical exercise is warranted.

Polio

Poliomyelitis (*polio*, for short) is a disease that was named in 1874 and is believed to affect the central nervous system.[2] According to the CDC, typical symptoms are flu-like, but severe cases can include paralysis, permanent disability, and death.[3]

When studying the illness in 1909, Drs. Simon Flexner and Paul Lewis claimed to experimentally demonstrate the transmission of polio. Their methodology, as summarized by authors Dawn Lester and David Parker, was as follows: "[Drs. Flexner and Lewis] produced paralysis by creating a concoction, which included the ground-up spinal cord from a 'polio' victim, that was injected into the brain of a living monkey. In order to prove 'transmission,' they extracted some of the fluid from the monkey's brain and injected that into the brain of another monkey. This series was continued through a number of monkeys. The fact that each subsequent monkey became paralyzed as a result of injections is claimed to provide the 'proof' of the infectious nature of the disease."[4]

In addition to the animal cruelty exhibited in the experiment, the methodology was problematic in its attempt to demonstrate a virus as the cause of illness—they transferred living tissue, not an isolated virus. They just assumed that a virus was in the tissue. Thus, their procedure was nowhere near the logical soundness of Koch's and Rivers's postulates.

And might it be the case that injecting spinal-cord tissue into monkey brains—by itself—causes illness? Control experiments involving the injection of other material into monkey brains would be necessary to scientifically demonstrate whether the injection procedure itself was causing symptoms.[5] Additionally, the injection method the doctors employed is unlike any natural means of alleged transmission. People who are believed to "catch" polio in real life aren't having their brains injected.[6]

(Note: These types of methodological issues are common among studies that attempt to demonstrate disease transmission. It should be simple to show that something so contagious is transmissible through normal and natural modes of contact. The symptoms of such diseases should also be easy to reproduce. And, given the widespread acceptance of germ theory, one would think there would already be an *abundance* of studies validating disease transmission for many, many "infectious diseases." But, as terrain theorists often argue, this is not the case.[7] The studies' methodologies are consistently flawed, and the researchers' treatment of animals is horrific.)

Yet, in spite of their study's shortcomings, Drs. Flexner and Lewis assumed that poliomyelitis was an infectious disease.[8] They hadn't even isolated a virus.

In fact, Christine Massey's aggregation of Freedom of Information requests reveals that the "polio virus" has never been properly isolated. Not only did the CDC fail to provide evidence but so did New Zealand's Ministry of Health, New Zealand's Institute of Environmental Science and Research, and various organizations in the United Kingdom (including Brighton and Hove City Council, Nottingham City Council/Public Health, Public Health at Rotherham Metropolitan Borough Council, Leicestershire County Council, Derby City Council, Hertfordshire County Council, Rutland County Council, London Borough of Bromley, Derbyshire County Council, Kirklees Council, Cheshire West and Chester Council, and London Borough of Lambeth.)[9]

An alternative perspective has emerged about polio, which links its typical symptoms to the use of toxic pesticides such as lead arsenate, BHC, and DDT.[10] DDT, in particular, was used heavily after being touted as "safe" in 1945 and was effective in killing bugs believed to carry malaria and typhus.[11] Prior to that, for instance, during the Great Depression of the 1930s, there were relatively few polio outbreaks. But after World War II, the disease seemed to appear every summer starting in 1945, largely among children. The vast majority of cases were diagnosed via symptoms alone.[12]

Cases of poliomyelitis spiked significantly into the early 1950s during the time of DDT use. Cornfields, fruit orchards, and even cows were drenched in DDT. Polio cases increased in the summer months—when DDT spraying was at its peak.[13]

Moreover, a belief had emerged that flies might be spreading polio, which provided further motivation to use DDT heavily. As noted on the History Channel's website: "Most middle-class Americans tended to associate disease with flies, dirt, and poverty....After World War II, Americans doused their neighborhoods, homes, and children with the highly toxic pesticide DDT in the hope of banishing polio....Yet, the number of cases grew larger each season."[14]

Endocrinologist Morton Biskind observed in 1953 that DDT itself had been known to cause symptoms that resemble those associated with polio. He stated: "Particularly relevant...are neglected studies...[from] the National Institutes of Health...which showed that DDT may produce degeneration of the anterior horn cells of the spinal cord in animals." Furthermore, he asserted, "When in 1945 DDT was released for use by the general public in the

United States and other countries, an impressive background of toxicological investigation had already showed beyond [a] doubt that this compound was dangerous for all animal life from insects to mammals. **It was even known by 1945 that DDT is stored in the body of mammals and appears in the milk.** With this foreknowledge, the series of catastrophic events that followed the most intensive campaign of mass poisoning in human history should not have surprised the experts."[15] [emphasis added]

Researcher Jim West compiled data in his book *DDT/Polio: Virology vs. Toxicology* (originally published in 1998 and updated in 2014), suggesting that the incidence of polio cases tracked closely with pesticide use from 1940 to 1970. That is, he showed a clear correlation between the incidence of polio and DDT use. But it wasn't just DDT. He also showed a link with *other pesticides* such as lead arsenate and BHC. At the very least, pesticide use was associated with the rise in polio, and the DDT craze might have caused a particularly significant spike in symptoms.[16] The figure that follows is a rendition of West's data analysis.[17]

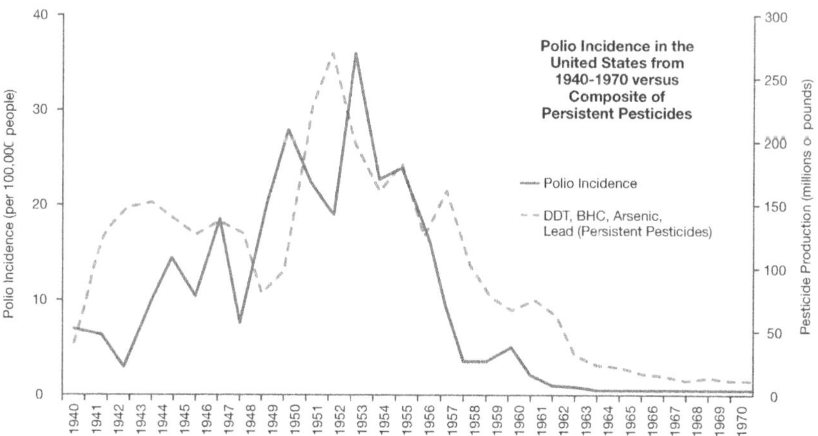

Re-created from Jim West's https://harvoa.org/polio/overview.htm. Per West's analysis, all production data is derived from U.S. Board of Transportation figures (Hayes and Laws, 1996); polio data is from U.S. Vital Statistics.

> **West also comments: "These four chemicals were not selected arbitrarily. These are representative of the major pesticides in use during the last major polio epidemic. They persist in the environment as neurotoxins that cause polio-like symptoms, polio-like physiology, and were dumped onto and into human food at dosage levels far above that approved by the FDA. They directly correlate with the incidence of various neurological diseases called 'polio' before 1965. They were utilized, according to Biskind, in the 'most intensive campaign of mass poisoning in known human history.'"**

Prior to the banning of DDT in the United States in 1972, its use was on the decline. As West notes, warning labels on packages were introduced, and DDT started to be used with much more caution. Also, Rachel Carson's 1962 book *Silent Spring* brought attention to the potential harms of pesticides.[18]

Polio cases peaked in 1952, but then began to dramatically decline in the late 1950s into the 1960s as pesticide use declined. This was *before* the introduction of Jonas Salk's polio vaccine in 1955.[19] Thus, while the vaccine is often credited as being the savior, there is another variable not often considered: reductions in the use of toxic pesticides.

Suzanne Humphries, MD, and Roman Bystrianyk lament in their book *Dissolving Illusions: Disease, Vaccines, and Forgotten History* (2013): "As of today, no programs have been funded to investigate or validate the scientific findings that implicate associations between chemicals like DDT and arsenic and the syndrome of poliomyelitis. Instead, the world is reliant upon blemished vintage research that was funded by the major medico-political powers of the first half of the 20th century."[20]

Similarly, in 1952, Ralph Scobey, MD, expressed his disappointment to the US House of Representatives: "For almost half a century, poliomyelitis investigations have been directed towards a supposed exogenous virus that enters the human body to cause the disease. The manner in which the Public Health Law is now stated, imposes only this type of investigation. No intensive studies have been made, on the other hand, to determine whether or not the so-called virus of poliomyelitis is an autochthonous [that is, indigenous] chemical substance that does not enter the human body at all, but simply results from an exogenous factor or factors, for example, a food poison."[21]

West adds: "In the works of [Dr. Scobey], I found that from ancient times to the early 20th century, the symptoms and physiology of paralytic poliomyelitis were often described as the results of *poisoning*. It wasn't until [the] mid-19th century that the word 'poliomyelitis' became the designation for the paralytic effects of severe poisoning and polio-like diseases assumed to be germ-caused."[22] [emphasis added]

West introduces a broader issue: that of *categorization*. This was clearly an issue with HIV/AIDS, and one might wonder if it's been an issue with "COVID-19" cases involving flu-like symptoms. Furthermore, given the problems associated with the gold-standard method of virus isolation discussed in chapter 2—and given that polio includes symptoms that could be misdiagnosed—might it be that accurate "polio" case counts are difficult to ascertain?

Although the medical establishment often talks about the dramatic global declines in polio in the modern era,[23] there are instances in which polio-like symptoms are flourishing. For instance, *The Hindu* reported in 2013: "Polio free does not mean paralysis free." The article mentions that in India there are many cases of "'acute flaccid paralysis' (AFP) that is symptomatic of polio....But AFP can also arise for other reasons, including infection by non-polio pathogens."[24] Could it be that AFP is just a different categorization of what has traditionally been called "polio"? Lester and Parker note that DDT was never banned in India, and it is being used there to fight malaria.[25]

Along similar lines, a study was published in *Reviews of Infectious Diseases* in 1984 titled "Nonpolio causes of polio-like paralytic syndromes." It states: "In a study of patients with suspected poliomyelitis, but from whom poliovirus was not isolated, a variety of causes of the paralysis was found...Chemical poisons, such as arsenic, triorthocresyl phosphate, and organophosphorus insecticides, were responsible for paralysis affecting groups of people."[26]

Again, one might wonder: Are these "nonpolio" conditions just simply artifacts of categorization? If polio isn't a viral disease, might all of the mentioned cases be the same thing, but they're just being labeled differently, which skews the data?

Defenders of the status quo dispute nonviral theories. For instance, the Associated Press published an article in 2023 titled "Experts say toxic pesticide DDT not linked to polio." The article quotes an email from a professor of immunology and microbiology at the University of Colorado: "Polio the disease is caused by the polio virus....DDT is a pesticide, so not clear [*sic*] how a pesticide could cause a viral infection."[27] Baked into this reasoning is the presupposition that what's known as "polio" is in fact caused by a virus.

Dr. Humphries and Bystrianyk add one more important paradox into the mix. Hygiene has sometimes been invoked as an explanation for polio, but the reasoning seems to break down because it's inconsistent. They write:

> By now it should be obvious that there was more to the "polio" story than a crippling virus and a world that was saved by a vaccine. Isn't it strange that the reasoning behind the polio epidemic in the United States in the 1940s was increased social hygiene? Filth, back then, was thought to be protective against polio! The explanation given was that babies in areas with better hygiene...were not exposed to wild virus early enough due to societal cleanliness and therefore did not develop early immunity.
>
> Today India is told that paralytic poliovirus infections are a result of poor societal hygiene. Such doublespeak demonstrates how the tenet changes to accommodate the vaccine agenda and deny the true causes of paralysis.[28]

Indeed, the reverence for vaccines seems to be a psychological hurdle for critical thinking here. Author Forrest Maready points to a parallel situation that is instructive in this regard. In Brazil in 2015, doctors began to see that babies were being born with small heads (a condition known as microcephaly). Maready notes: "Despite locals pointing to the release of genetically modified mosquitoes or the aggressive pesticide spraying they had been recently subjected to, authorities were sure they had found the cause[:]...a microbe transmitted by [a] mosquito bite called the Zika virus."[29] There was a rush to develop a vaccine. But by 2016, birth defects had subsided, and the vaccine rush quieted with it. As Maready writes in his book *The Moth in the Iron Lung: A Biography of Polio* (2018):

> Although the timeline is condensed, the Zika story closely mirrors what happened with polio....The possibility of environmental causes as a contributing factor are largely ignored by health officials....
>
> [However,] there is a distinct difference between [polio and Zika]. With poliomyelitis, vaccines were licensed and began to be administered. The vaccines—despite their admitted inefficacy and late arrival to the scene—were declared a complete success....
>
> Zika had no such program. If it did, there is little doubt that the fall in microcephaly rates would be attributed to the success of the vaccine. Claims to the contrary would be brushed aside....A search for the true cause of the spike in microcephaly that year in Brazil would be scoffed at as the wild hunt of a conspiracy theorist."[30]

Maready summarizes the situation well: "Humans prefer a heroic story rather than one of dismal failure....The audacious tale of how the polio vaccine saved us from harm is so ingrained into cultural lore, it feels wrong to dispute it—indeed, many are attacked for daring to question a single detail. Because of this, the story has lived on."[31]

Such a story also appeals to the reductionistic mindset of allopathic medicine that likes to simplify disease to a single cause such as a "virus," which enables a single cure such as a "vaccine." As Maready writes: "The search for a single causative agent planted a deep seed within the psyches of scientists and physicians everywhere—the idea that paralytic poliomyelitis was caused by a single virus, despite all evidence to the contrary. Unfortunately, modern science has not escaped this same tunnel vision."[32]

SARS

Severe acute respiratory syndrome (SARS) first appeared in November 2002 in Guangdong, China.[33] The syndrome was alleged to be caused by a virus dubbed SARS-CoV-1, the so-called predecessor to SARS-CoV-2.

The WHO states: "SARS is an airborne virus and can spread through small droplets of saliva in a similar way to the cold and influenza. It was the first severe and readily transmissible new disease to emerge in the 21st century and showed a clear capacity to spread along the routes of international air travel. SARS can also be spread indirectly via surfaces that have been touched by someone who is infected with the virus."[34]

Symptoms included fever, shortness of breath, and hypoxemia (low blood-oxygen levels). By 2005, the virus "disappeared." There were roughly 8,000 cases, and the fatality rate was, alarmingly, around 10 percent.[35]

The authors of *Virus Mania*, Engelbrecht et al., note that Guangdong, China, is a site where "for $1.50 a day, locals disassemble computers, monitors, and printers with their bare hands, endangering their own health and the environment." In particular, Guiyu, Guangdong, became a "booming center of e-waste since the mid-1990s....Workers empty toner cartridges from laser printers all day long without protective masks, breathing in fine carbon dust. Others...dip circuit boards into baths of liquid lead to separate and collect the soldering materials with which the memory chips and processors are attached to the plates. Unprotected, they are exposed to toxic fumes....A lot of garbage is simply burned up or dumped onto rice fields, irrigation facilities, or into waterways."[36] Toxicity, therefore, should be considered as at least a *possible* factor in the SARS scare.

Uncovering the root cause of "SARS" is also complicated because of problems with the isolation of the alleged virus itself. In 2005, Engelbrecht et al. wrote to the Robert Koch Institute of Germany requesting studies showing the isolation of the alleged SARS virus, that the virus causes disease, and that other factors like toxins and malnutrition aren't at least co-factors. No studies were given to them in response that met the authors' criteria.[37] Similarly, according to the Freedom of Information requests aggregated by Christine Massey, organizations around the world (including the CDC) have failed to provide evidence of a properly isolated SARS virus or common-cold coronavirus.[38]

The alleged discovery of SARS as the primary causative agent of disease is often believed to be shown in a July 2003 paper in *The Lancet* medical journal, titled "Newly discovered coronavirus as the primary cause of severe acute respiratory syndrome."[39] **However, an examination of its methodologies illustrates problems seen repeatedly in studies claiming to demonstrate that germs cause disease.** Dr. Samantha Bailey comprehensively summarizes the study, its weaknesses, and what should have been done instead:

> Firstly, [the researchers] took a sample from a SARS victim and then produced a cellular culture in the lab....Monkeys were then "infected" [when researchers squirted] this mixture into their tracheas, noses, and eyes. On the second, fourth, and sixth days, the monkeys were anesthetized with ketamine, an anesthetic known for its hallucinogenic properties. Blood samples were taken...and smears were obtained from the throat, nose, mouth, and anus. The monkeys were all killed for autopsies after just six days.
>
> Three of the monkeys became lethargic after two or three days. On the fourth day, two developed temporary rashes. Only one monkey had any breathing difficulties, while three showed non-advancing tissue damage to the lungs. The lymph nodes near the trachea and the spleen were larger than normal in these three monkeys.

The other organs all appeared normal under microscopic examination.

There are some glaring weaknesses with this study. Firstly, the monkeys' illnesses were not typical of SARS. Only one monkey had breathing issues, and there was no mention of any of them having a cough or fever, which are some of the key features of SARS. And none of the monkeys became critically unwell or died from SARS. They were all euthanized by the researchers.

Secondly, the paper claimed to identify coronavirus particles in monkey tissue on electron microscopy. But many different virus-sized particles are part of the cell culture. So without particle purification it's impossible to know exactly what they were.

There seems to have been a lot of confusion about isolation and purification. Purification means...we just have the alleged [viral particles] by themselves....So if it's not purified, then there will be other viral-sized particles in the material which may appear in the electron micrograph image and may also contribute other genetic fragments.

Thirdly, injecting 4 milliliters of culture solution directly into a small animal's trachea is a way to cause a lung reaction. Given that these little primates weigh around 5 or 7 kilograms, it would be the equivalent of injecting, say, 50 milliliters or almost 2 fluid ounces of culture solution into a human subject. Introducing that amount of material directly into the trachea has the potential to flow into the lungs and cause reactive changes....

On this note, it is also unclear what conclusions you can draw from injecting viral cultures directly into an animal's upper respiratory system and then a few days later finding it in the lower respiratory system....This has not helped confirm Koch's postulates as [the authors] claimed [in their paper]....

There was [also] a fatal flaw with regards to the study's design. There was no control group. Stressful physical containment and the procedures themselves like being anesthetized with ketamine multiple times have definite effects on animals, including potential histological changes in their tissues....No control=not scientific. A control is necessary to exclude the possibility that experimental findings may arise because of suspected or unsuspected factors unrelated to one's hypothesis.

How should it have been done? Test and control monkeys should have been matched in every way. This includes: sharing similar demographics, cages, food handling, care, medical history, clinical laboratory, and radiological findings. The only difference being that the material administered to the control group would be minus the [SARS virus]-isolate obtained from [the patient] who died of SARS. The control and test subject experiments must run in parallel using exactly the same methods. And to minimize bias, the experimenter must be blind to the identity of both groups.

Since there is no proof that the material given to the monkeys was [the] purified [virus], it is simply impossible to conclude that the effects observed in the four monkeys were specifically due to the [the virus] alone. It is possible that the control monkeys given the same material devoid of [the virus] may have suffered the same effects.

Additionally, these SARS-animal studies do not produce either aerosol or real-world host-to-host transmission of the alleged pathogen. If we are dealing with such a highly infectious agent, shouldn't we just introduce one infected animal into a contained space, and then the others will soon become infected too? Don't forget that the *New York Times* claimed that SARS can be so explosive that scores of family members and health workers can be infected from a cough

> from one patient. Shouldn't re-creating these terribly infectious so-called super spreaders be a slam dunk?[40] [emphasis added]

So this study failed to identify an isolated, purified virus, didn't use proper controls, and didn't demonstrate natural transmission. Given the intense scare associated with SARS, the study's weak design is startling.

Another often-referenced study is from *Nature* in 2003, titled "Koch's postulates fulfilled for SARS virus."[41] In order to try to meet Koch's postulates, first the virus has to be isolated. The paper's "proof" of isolation was to cite other papers that claimed to have isolated SARS-CoV-1, and then used a cell-culture soup for their experiment.

Furthermore, this paper was submitted by a mainstream scientist in response to a challenge issued by Dr. Thomas Cowan more recently (in August 2023). Dr. Cowan had a specific request: he asked for any properly controlled studies—ever conducted—that demonstrated germ-based contagion via a very basic method. He wanted studies showing *that sick people or animals make well people or animals sick.*[42] This is alleged to happen in the real world all the time via germ-based contagion. So shouldn't there be an abundance of such studies, for every allegedly contagious disease?

Dr. Cowan provided a commonsense critique of the 2003 *Nature* study that was submitted in response to his challenge, and it's illustrative of broader problems with studies alleging to demonstrate contagion. The method used in the study was to inoculate two macaque monkeys with a cell-culture soup that was assumed to carry the virus (because it included fluids from someone who died of SARS). As a reminder, cell cultures typically have antibiotics, monkey kidney cells, and a variety of other substances—and the fluids of a sick person are added to it. Dr. Cowan notes that the design is problematic for his challenge because there weren't any sick people or animals in the study, as he had requested. Only the fluids from a sick person were part of the study because the monkeys were inoculated with a cell-culture soup that included fluids from a sick person.

As Dr. Cowan puts it: "This is so far removed from anything that anybody has any experience with....In other words, in all my years of medicine, nobody came to me and said, 'Tom, I was doing fine and then somebody inoculated me with the results of a cell culture, and I've been sick as a dog ever since.' That never once happened. This has no relation to any phenomenon that anybody would ever see in nature."[43] [emphasis added]

Finally, the many problems discussed with studies on SARS-CoV-1 also apply to the more recent SARS-CoV-2, which was discussed in chapter 2. In contrast to the study just mentioned, which claimed to have fulfilled Koch's postulates for SARS-CoV-1, the following study said it didn't for SARS-CoV-2. It was one of the early studies claiming to have identified a novel coronavirus—published in the *New England Journal of Medicine* in January 2020—shortly before the panic and lockdowns began. **And it explicitly states: "Our study does not fulfill Koch's postulates."**[44] **Recall from chapter 3 that in 2003, the WHO stated that "conclusive identification of a causative [agent] must meet all criteria of the so-called Koch's postulate [*sic*]."**[45] [emphasis added]

Additionally, one of the paper's authors even revealed that the electron-microscope images taken in the study had "an image of sedimented virus particles, not purified ones."[46]

Without first establishing an isolated, purified virus, said virus cannot be shown to be the cause of disease.

The Spanish Flu (1918–1919)

The Spanish flu was the deadliest pandemic in world history, alleged to have been responsible for as many as 50 million deaths worldwide.[47] Milton Rosenau, MD, conducted experiments—detailed in August 1919 in the *Journal of the American Medical Association*—which included numerous failed attempts to show that the disease was contagious. And in some parts of the experiment, he attempted much more natural transmission modes than are seen in other studies.

In collaboration with the US Navy and Public Health Service, Dr. Rosenau conducted his studies with one hundred Navy volunteers. The first group of experiments was conducted at Gallops Island in the Boston Harbor Islands.

The experimenters began by administering "a pure culture of bacillus of influenza, Pfeiffer's bacillus, in a rather moderate amount, into the nostrils of a few of [the] volunteers."[48] None of them got sick.

Next, large quantities of various strains of the germ "were sprayed with an atomizer into the nose and into the eyes, and back into the throat, while the volunteers were breathing in."[49] Dr. Rosenau noted, "We used some billions of these organisms, according to our estimated counts, on each one of the volunteers [who] were sprayed." None of them got sick.

Next, "mucous secretions of the mouth and nose and throat and bronchi"[50]—taken from people sick with Spanish flu—were sprayed into volunteers' nostrils, throats, and eyes. None of them got sick.

The experimenters wondered if they couldn't get volunteers sick because there was too much time in between extracting the diseased material and administering it to the volunteers (roughly four hours). So they reduced the interval to one hour and forty minutes, and then administered the diseased material into volunteers' nostrils, throats, and eyes. None of them got sick.

Wondering if the salt solution used in the administration of diseased material might have impacted the results, the experimenters transferred the material directly from nose to nose and throat to throat using small sticks with cotton swabs on the end. None of the healthy people got sick. Dr. Rosenau clarified, "When I say none of them took sick in any way, I mean that after receiving the material, they were then isolated on Gallops Island. Their temperature was taken three times a day and carefully examined, of course, and under constant medical supervision they were held for one full week before they were released, and perhaps used again for some other experiment."[51]

The experimenters then tried direct injections. First, they took blood from sick patients and injected it into the healthy volunteers. None of them got sick. Then they extracted "a lot of [diseased] mucous material from the upper respiratory tract"[52] and injected it into healthy volunteers. None of them got sick.

The next attempt was a more natural mode: human contact. Dr. Rosenau explained the methodology:

> The volunteer was led up to the bedside of the patient; he was introduced. He sat down alongside the bed of the patient. They shook hands, and by instructions, he got as close as he conveniently could, and they talked for five minutes. At the end of the five minutes, the patient breathed out as hard as he could, while the volunteer, muzzle to muzzle (in accordance with his instructions, about 2 inches between the two), received this expired breath, and at the same time was breathing in as the patient breathed out. This they repeated five times, and they did it fairly faithfully in almost all of the instances.
>
> **After they had done this five times, the patient coughed directly into the face of the volunteer, face to face, five different times.**
>
> I may say that the volunteers were perfectly splendid about carrying out the technic [*sic*] of these experiments. They did it with a high idealism. They were inspired with the thought that they might help others. They went through the program in a splendid spirit. After our volunteer had had this sort of contact with the patient, talking and chatting and shaking hands with him for five minutes, and receiving his breath five times, and then his cough five times directly in his face, he moved to the next patient whom we had selected, and repeated this, and so on, until this volunteer had had that sort of contact with **ten different cases of influenza**, in

> different stages of the disease, mostly fresh cases, none of them more than three days old.[53] [emphasis added]

Dr. Rosenau added: "We will remember that each one of the ten volunteers had that sort of intimate contact with each one of the ten different influenza patients. They were watched carefully for seven days—**and none of them took sick in any way**."[54] [emphasis added]

The experimenters then temporarily suspended their work and later tried again, repeating the methods of the early experiments, at Portsmouth. This time, about half the number of volunteers exposed to diseased material had a fever and sore throat. However, Dr. Rosenau noted, "All the clinicians who saw these cases in consultation agreed with us that they were ordinary cases of sore throat."[55] Remember: the Spanish flu was supposed to be the deadliest pandemic in world history.

In another instance at Portsmouth, none of the volunteers got sick. However, one experimenter—who collected material from the volunteers and had been in "intimate contact with the disease" for months—got sick with "a clinical attack of influenza...although he had escaped all the rest of the outbreak."[56]

Dr. Rosenau stated in conclusion:

> I think we must be very careful not to draw any positive conclusions from negative results of this kind. Many factors must be considered. Our volunteers may not have been susceptible. They may have been immune. They had been exposed, as all the rest of the people had been exposed to the disease, although they gave no clinical history of an attack.
>
> **Dr. McCoy, who with Dr. Richey, did a similar series of experiments on Goat Island, San Francisco, used volunteers who, so far as known, had not been exposed to the outbreak at all, also had negative results, that is, they were unable to reproduce the disease. Perhaps**

> **there are factors, or a factor, in the transmission of influenza that we do not know.**
>
> **As a matter of fact, we entered the outbreak with a notion that we knew the cause of the disease, and were quite sure we knew how it was transmitted from person to person. Perhaps, if we have learned anything, it is that we are not quite sure what we know about the disease.**[57] [emphasis added]

Dr. Rosenau and his colleagues conducted additional studies and got similar results.[58]

These eye-opening experiments certainly challenge the traditional narrative about the disease. However, in 1997, a paper claimed to have isolated the virus from the preserved lung tissue of a soldier who died in 1918, and additional papers claiming to have isolated the virus were published in 2005. The media spun this with sensationalism: "US researchers revive old killer virus."[59] As Engelbrecht et al. note: "Even if headlines suggest this, the fact is that a virus with complete genetic material (genome) has never been discovered. Lung tissue samples were simply taken from several corpses from that time….Researchers had not proven that the genetic material they found really belongs to a pathogenic 'old killer virus.' With many samples, the tests even came out 'negative.' The whole thing, then, is pure speculation."[60]

But *something* was resulting in huge death counts during the Spanish-flu era. Many patients were reporting blood in the lungs—which, incidentally, was a symptom associated with the smallpox vaccine at the time. Mass vaccination, up to twenty-four vaccines per person, was reported.[61]

Eleanor McBean, PhD, also expressed this perspective based on her own experience during the Spanish flu. She wrote in her 1977 book, *Swine Flu Expose*:

> One thing is certain—the 1918 Spanish influenza was a vaccine-induced disease caused by extreme body

poisoning from the conglomeration of many different vaccines....

That pandemic dragged on for two years, kept alive with the addition of more poison drugs administered by the doctors who tried to suppress the symptoms. **As far as I could find out, the flu hit only the vaccinated. Those who had refused the shots escaped the flu. My family had refused all the vaccinations so we remained well all the time....**

When the flu was at its peak, all the stores were closed as well as the schools, businesses—even the hospital, as the doctors and nurses had been vaccinated too and were down with the flu. No one was on the streets. It was like a ghost town. We seemed to be the only family which didn't get the flu; so my parents went from house to house doing what they could to look after the sick, as it was impossible to get a doctor then. If it were possible for germs, bacteria, virus, or bacilli to cause disease, they had plenty of opportunity to attack my parents when they were spending many hours a day in the sick rooms. But they didn't get the flu, and they didn't bring any germs home to attack us children and cause anything. None of our family had the flu—not even a sniffle—and it was in the winter with deep snow on the ground....

There was seven times more disease among the vaccinated soldiers than among the unvaccinated civilians, and the diseases were those they had been vaccinated against. One soldier who had returned from overseas in 1912 told me that the army hospitals were filled with cases of infantile paralysis, and he wondered why grown men should have an infant disease. Now, we know that paralysis is a common after-effect of vaccine poisoning. Those at home didn't get the paralysis until after the worldwide vaccination campaign in 1918.[62] [emphasis added]

Engelbrecht et al. also cite Anne Riley Hale's 1935 book, *Medical Voodoo*, in which the author states: "As everyone knows, the world has never witnessed such an orgy of vaccination and inoculation of every description that was inflicted by army-camp doctors upon soldiers of the [First] World War."[63]

An additional possibility is suggested by Arthur Firstenberg in his book *The Invisible Rainbow* (2020): electrical pollution. **As the world was industrializing, perhaps increased electricity caused more health problems than people realized (and perhaps that's still true today).**

Firstenberg uses the term *acute electrical illness*. He writes: "During the 1918–1919 pandemic, monkeys and baboons perished in great numbers in South Africa, sheep in northwest England, horses in France, moose in northern Canada, and buffalo in Yellowstone. There is no mystery there. We're not catching flu from animals, nor they from us. **If influenza is caused by electromagnetic conditions in the atmosphere, then it affects all living things at the same time."[64]** [emphasis added]

This is a particularly relevant idea if the human body has a greater electric-like aspect than is acknowledged by allopathic medicine, such as a biofield (more on this in chapter 7).

Avian Flu (also known as bird flu, or H5NI)

According to the WHO, the avian flu affects birds and is not normally known to infect humans.[65] But it apparently *can* affect humans, and there have been a number of scares reported in the media.

Again, Engelbrecht et al. reached out to various publications asking for basic things: studies proving that the virus exists, causes disease, and jumps to the human species. The authors report that various outlets "could not name a single study."[66] Then, they then reached out to the Friedrich-Loeffler-Institut (FLI), which they had been told was in possession of "pure H5N1 viral cultures." The FLI sent the authors four studies, but again those studies did not offer the proof that they were seeking, and they also didn't receive an electron micrograph of the purified virus.[67]

One study that the FLI sent to the authors described a young boy who died after facing progressive pneumonia. He was treated with what the authors believe were toxic medications, and then was said to have "died during the late phase of the [H5N1] disease after intensive treatment with antiviral drugs." Additionally, H5N1 could not be detected in any of the patient's diseased organs, which the researchers shrugged off as an "enigma" (rather than considering that perhaps H5N1 wasn't the cause of disease, and maybe the toxic medications made his condition worse).[68]

Additionally, Engelbrecht et al. comment that for avian flu, like so many other viruses, the PCR test—an indirect way to validate a virus's existence—was problematic.[69] As discussed in chapter 1, Dr. Kary Mullis, the Nobel Prize–winning inventor of the PCR test, said that PCR can be used to find *anything*. And furthermore, if the virus itself hadn't been properly isolated, whatever genetic material the PCR was working with couldn't be directly tied to the alleged virus.

Although the WHO claims that more than 150 people died of avian flu from 2003 to 2006, Engelbrecht et al. remark: "There is no direct evidence for the theory that H5N1 was the killer.... The reports [of deaths] allow completely different possibilities... as plausible explanations. For example, that some of the victims were suffering from cold symptoms of an unknown source and they simply had the bad luck to fall into the hands of medical professionals who turned out to be H5N1 hunters."[70]

These anomalies, in addition to those discussed regarding the Spanish flu, perhaps explain why Ben Killingley, MD, et al. wrote in a 2012 *Journal of Infectious Diseases* article: "Influenza transmission in humans remains poorly understood."[71]

Smallpox

Smallpox is commonly believed to be a contagious viral disease that causes a distinctive skin rash, and according to the CDC, it causes death in three out of ten people.[72]

In the United States, there haven't been any outbreaks since 1949, and no "naturally occurring" cases have occurred since 1979. Vaccines are believed to have eradicated the illness. The initial version of the vaccine was famously developed in 1796 by English doctor William Jenner.[73] According to the CDC, smallpox has existed for at least 3,000 years, resulting in the deaths of countless people throughout human history.[74]

However, smallpox is one of the "viruses" for which Christine Massey submitted a Freedom of Information request. She asked for evidence that the smallpox virus has been properly isolated. The CDC's January 5, 2022, response to her request stated that it was unable to provide any such studies or reports.[75]

In 1901, a Wisconsin physician named Matthew Joseph Rodermund personally challenged the notion that smallpox is a contagious disease.[76] Dr. Rodermund's account was documented by J. W. Hodge, MD, in 1902. As Dr. Rodermund told the story, he entered a family's home with a woman who had smallpox and asserted that "you can't take the disease from another." He further reported: "Then to show [the family] that this was true, I broke open several of the large pustules on her face and arms and took the pus out of them and smeared it all over my face, hands, beard and clothes, and at the same time remarked that I would now go home to dinner."[77] He went home and didn't mention the event to his family, and then went to his office where he shook hands with an old friend, writing of the event: "I had entirely forgotten that I was covered with smallpox....During the same afternoon, I touched the faces of several persons in my office while treating their eyes and fitting their glasses....The same afternoon, I was at the Business Men's Club where I mingled and played cards."[78] He noted: "I would never have gone to the club rooms if I'd had the least idea that my actions would ever be known....**I have done**

similar acts dozens of times during the past fifteen years and have in each instance watched the results, and not the slightest harm has ever been done to anyone."[79] [emphasis added]

Dr. Rodermund went about his normal routine the next day—without washing himself. He wore the same clothes and interacted with many more people. The following day, he washed his hands and face, for the first time in forty-six and a half hours, and was greeted at his office by reporters who'd heard about what he'd done when he visited the smallpox patient. One of the patient's neighbors had seen Dr. Rodermund leave the home and asked the local health officer whether the family had changed doctors.

Knowing that the cat was out of the bag, Dr. Rodermund told "the exact truth."[80] The next day he was quarantined and guarded by police officers. He then escaped quarantine, driving miles from home and taking a train, but was arrested on the way back and placed in quarantine again for several days. The *New York Times* even picked up the story.[81]

Dr. Rodermund summarized the situation:

> The sanctimonious frauds and deceivers of the public (doctors) tried in every way, shape, and manner to trace a case of smallpox to my actions, but to no avail. **Even after I had exposed 50,000 people, and rubbed my pus-covered hands over thirty-seven faces, they could find nothing against me....**
>
> Why has not one of the thousands of these medical scoundrels, murderers, and deceivers ever turned up to win the prize, which reads as follows: "One thousand dollars will be given to anyone who can prove that disease is contagious."...
>
> The doctors knew that by superstition the people best be held. Then, I want to ask you, are not the people more to blame than the doctors?
>
> **More than half the public do not believe in contagion, but they lack the courage to say so.** Discussion

> and argument will never change the present conditions. They never settle a question where a powerful body of men have law and money on their side. A powerful public sentiment, combined with true knowledge, is the only remedy. As long as you drowse in your old superstitions, these murderers will continue to ruin your constitutions for the money there is in it.[82] [emphasis added]

Dr. Rodermund's experience suggests that the entire narrative of this disease needs to at least be reconsidered—including accounts of smallpox that were reported hundreds of years ago.

For instance, one of the most well-known stories about smallpox is that the settlers of the "New World" traveled across the Atlantic Ocean and brought over the disease from Europe. This allegedly contributed to the genocide of the native people. Settlers are said to have engaged in "biological warfare" by giving the natives their blankets that were contaminated with smallpox, while the settlers themselves were unaffected.[83] In other words, the settlers were believed to be asymptomatic carriers. Authors Dawn Lester and David Parker note the oddity in this often-accepted concept: on the one hand, the settlers are claimed to have been immune, which seems to imply that they wouldn't have been harboring the deadly germs due to their "antibodies"—but if they had smallpox, they wouldn't be immune.[84]

Lester and Parker point to factors other than smallpox that can explain the genocide, however. They cite books such as *American Holocaust: Conquest of the New World* (1993), by David Stannard, PhD; and Eduardo Galeano's *Open Veins of Latin America* (1997).

The Spanish settlers were enamored with the golden jewelry of the natives, so they confiscated some and forced the natives to work in mines to get more. The conditions were brutal: the ventilation was poor, and the natives were breathing in poisonous gases. This could have resulted in untold deaths that aren't often accounted for.[85] Furthermore, the British used tactics of starvation and massacre with the natives.

Lester and Parker remark: "The medical establishment has a clear vested interest in perpetuating the myth that it was the 'germs' that killed many millions of people who had no immunity to the diseases the germs are alleged to cause."[86]

Poor sanitation is another factor to address when rethinking the smallpox story. Walter Hawden, MD, wrote in 1923: "One fact stands out pre-eminently in every part of [the] world where smallpox has appeared—namely, it has been invariably associated with insanitary and unhygienic conditions....It has followed in the wake of filth, poverty, wars, pestilences, famines, and general insanitation, in all ages."[87]

In 1957, Dr. Eleanor McBean elaborated on the types of sanitation improvements that began in 1800, which in her mind, are responsible for the decline in smallpox: "(1) sewage disposal; (2) cleaning of streets, back yards, stables, etc.; (3) improvements of roads so that fresh vegetables, milk, and other vital foods could be transported rapidly to cities and distributed while still fresh; (4) the water supply was improved and protected from contamination; and (5) housing projects were built out in the suburbs to relieve congestion of [the] population in the cities." She also felt that improved nutrition habits, beginning in 1840, played a role. As she bluntly put it: "The simple fact that we have less smallpox now than we did 200 years ago does not prove that vaccination caused this decline."[88]

Lester and Parker also note that in the 19th century, Cleveland, Ohio, and the British town of Leicester focused on sanitation and also rejected vaccination (at a time when smallpox vaccines were ubiquitous). In both cities, smallpox disappeared.[89] These "anomalies" damage the allopathic narrative that the smallpox vaccine was the savior it is often believed to have been. Further data is presented by Dr. Humphries and Bystrianyk, which led them to conclude that "compulsory vaccination laws did nothing to curb the problem of smallpox."[90]

An additional relevant factor is that the medicines prescribed to treat smallpox were themselves toxic. Until the early 20th century, mercury, arsenic, and antimony were given to people afflicted with smallpox. Gerard Buchwald, MD (1920–2009), even suggested that smallpox started to go away when these toxic treatments were prohibited.[91]

Along similar lines, for some time, leprosy and syphilis were treated with mercury ointments. Lester and Parker note that mercury poisoning can lead to a shedding of the skin—a symptom that could have been confused with smallpox (and leprosy and syphilis).[92]

A 2020 study published in *Current Problems in Pediatric and Adolescent Health Care* supports this notion. The paper's title is instructive: "All that glitters is not gold: Mercury poisoning in a family mimicking an infectious illness." The authors describe patients who were "heavily exposed to elemental mercury that was spilled in their home and then vacuumed." They further comment: "**Clinically significant elemental mercury toxicity can resemble an infectious illness.** Severe morbidity and mortality can be prevented if heavy metal poisoning is considered early."[93] [emphasis added]

These various hypotheses collectively challenge the allopathic notion that smallpox is a contagious virus. Instead, the symptoms associated with what's known as "smallpox" might reflect the body's reaction to, and attempt to cleanse itself from, various forms of toxicity.

Chicken Pox

In a 2023 article in *Clinical Dermatology*, Amber Czinn and Leonard Hoenig state: "The word 'pox' indicated, during the late 15th century, a disease characterized by eruptive sores. When an outbreak of syphilis began in Europe during that time, it was called by many names, including the French term 'la grosse verole' ('the great pox'), to distinguish it from smallpox, which was termed 'la petite verole' ('the small pox'). Chicken pox was initially confused with smallpox until 1767, when the English physician William

Heberden (1710–1801) provided a detailed description of chicken pox, differentiating it from smallpox."[94]

This historical narrative implies that these allegedly contagious "poxviruses" are distinct. However, one might wonder if the distinctions are artificial and misleading—and that these allegedly separate diseases actually reflect a spectrum of bodily detoxification responses that are unrelated to an alleged pathogen.

With regard to chicken pox, the disease has certainly been correlated with close contact—so much so that parents have taken their children to "chicken-pox parties" so that the kids can get the illness (and get it over with). But people sharing an environment can get sick for reasons other than a viral infection.

A more fundamental problem is that the chicken pox virus "isolation" experiments are lacking. Dr. Samantha Bailey comments: "Throughout the chicken pox literature, the same claim is made that the disease is caused by the highly contagious varicella virus. But nobody cites an original paper where this was established.... It's not apparent to me that there are any original scientific studies that the causative agent of chicken pox is a virus." She also cites studies that *allege* to have isolated the virus, but not surprisingly they use the standard (flawed) cell-culture method discussed in chapter 2.[95]

Additionally, in 1919, Alfred Hess, MD, questioned the transmissibility of chicken pox (as well as measles). He made the following comments in the *Journal of the American Medical Association* on October 18, 1919:

> I have just read the abstract in The Journal (Oct. 4, 1919, p. 1086) of Sellards' article on "The Insusceptibility of Man to Inoculation with Blood from Measles Patients" (Bull. Johns Hopkins Hosp. 30:257 [Sept.] 1919).
>
> It is remarkable that Sellards was unable to produce this highly infectious disease by means of the blood or the nasal secretion of infected individuals. Not long ago, however, **I had a similar experience with varicella**

> [chicken pox]....**Thus we are confronted with two diseases—the two most infectious of the endemic diseases in this part of the world—which we are unable to transmit artificially from man to man. The result was most surprising in regard to chicken pox, and if the same rule holds good for measles, it would seem as if a basic principle must be involved. Evidently in our experiments, we do not, as we believe, pursue nature's mode of transmission; either we fail to carry over the virus, or the path to infection is quite different from what it is commonly thought to be.**[96] [emphasis added]

So if chicken pox doesn't come from a contagious virus, how would we explain what happens at chicken-pox parties? For one, not everyone gets sick at such parties, which raises questions about the viral contagion model generally. If it's so contagious, why wouldn't *everyone* get sick? Is there a definitive explanation? Dr. Bailey notes, "I've seen plenty of cases where only one person in a household gets chicken pox, including when there are several other children in proximity."[97]

There could also be an element of an energetic "resonance" between sick people in the same place. This is a concept that ties in with the forthcoming discussion about consciousness in chapters 6 and 7. Alternative theories like this require a total rethinking of the nature of reality itself, which opens up possibilities not considered by allopathic medicine. Similarly, Dr. Thomas Cowan and Sally Fallon Morell speculate that so-called sexually transmitted diseases might actually relate to factors such as resonance rather than an infectious pathogen. In this regard, the "contagion" is on an energetic level of some sort; it's not a biological germ.[98] On a related topic, Dr. Bailey notes that there is a lack of evidence that herpes is a contagious virus—and wonders instead whether the blisters reflect the body's attempt to rid itself of toxins. She also comments that the blisters might result from an intense emotional state such as stress (that is, one's state of consciousness can manifest through physical symptoms).[99] Hypotheses like these would need to be investigated much further to see if there's any validity to them—but the majority of allopathic medicine's attention, and dollars, are focused elsewhere.[100]

Additionally, consider the fact that female roommates sometimes synchronize their menstrual cycles.[101] Is this because of chemical emissions from the body known as "pheromones"? Or is there something more "energetic" at play? Also consider that women's menstrual cycles can synchronize with the moon, as discussed in a 2021 article in *Science Advances* (a peer-reviewed journal).[102] Suffice it to say that we have a lot to learn about biology.

Moreover, it's worth noting that chicken-pox parties are typically among children who are of a similar age, and one might wonder if there is a hormonal element that should be evaluated.[103] Dr. Andrew Kaufman provides another hypothesis, which is that perhaps chicken pox is a "purging" that enables the skin to grow properly. That is, maybe it's part of the development of the broader musculoskeletal system.[104] Dr. Cowan and Morell note that there might be other benefits to getting chicken pox, even though the mechanism isn't understood. They describe the illness as "a universal way for children to live a long life. Children who experience chicken pox have less disease (and especially less cancer) than do children who haven't had chicken pox. The same holds for measles, mumps, and most childhood 'infectious' diseases."[105]

In fact, chicken pox has an extremely low death rate. Dr. Bailey notes that even though the CDC markets the chicken-pox vaccine as an important development that has lowered deaths, death rates were already trending down before the introduction of the vaccine. She comments, "If you look at the tiny number of mortalities, two out of the three children that died between 2012 and 2016 had severe underlying diseases such as leukemia, and one out of the two had been vaccinated."[106]

On a related note, shingles deserves a brief mention. Per the CDC's definition: "Shingles is caused by the varicella-zoster virus (VZV), the same virus that causes chicken pox. Once a person has chicken pox, the virus stays in their body. The virus can reactivate later in life and cause shingles."[107] The CDC does not cite any scientific evidence for this claim.

Dr. Cowan feels that this thinking is a form of "inventive reasoning" that commonly occurs when a presupposition is held as immutable, even when it hasn't been established—which then forces people to make things up out of thin air to explain related phenomena. And yet those explanations are held as truth, which leads people to believe a cascade of unsubstantiated, superstitious stories.

With regard to shingles, Dr. Cowan explains:

> You have to find the organism, the chicken pox virus,… you have to isolate it, which has never been properly done, and then you have to show that only the virus causes chicken pox….[So mainstream doctors] invent a story—they don't actually demonstrate that the story is true—and when there are flaws in the story [they invent new things around it]. In other words [there is a belief that] you only get chicken pox once, and then you're immune for life. And then, whoops, you seem to get the same illness again later with a slightly different manifestation, so then you have to invent another story to account for that, which is that your immune system got weak, and that led the virus to erupt, and it's called [shingles]—none of which has ever been substantiated.[108]

Modern allopathic medicine is likely filled with many such stories that are treated as truth but haven't been scientifically established. Therefore, they are simply invented to preserve existing dogma, and the public repeats the stories as if they are established facts.

Hepatitis

Hepatitis refers to inflammation of the liver, and according to the CDC, it is often caused by a virus.[109] Dr. Samamtha Bailey notes that, historically, recovery from liver-related illnesses involved a review of lifestyle factors and even spending months at health retreats for recovery. Today, on the other hand, most doctors will give patients a blood test to look for a virus. The same problem emerges that we've seen elsewhere. In Dr. Bailey's words: "Where is the virus?"[110]

She references a 2002 paper in the *BMJ* stating that alcohol consumption is a key factor for the condition, and the "virus" doesn't have a big impact on all-cause mortality. Claus Köhnlein, MD, one of the coauthors of *Virus Mania*, responded to the *BMJ* paper shortly after it was published:

> They all found low liver-related morbidity and mortality rates, except in people who drink excessive alcohol. We don't need a virus to explain this.
>
> Going back to the roots of Hepatitis C, we find in *The Lancet*, March 1978 (Alter et al.), that there was no transmissible agent found. Instead, blood from a patient with...hepatitis was inoculated into five chimps. Three of the animals developed a transient elevation of aminotransferases [a metric of liver damage] around week 15. A control animal was kept in a separate room. The possibility of immune reactions against foreign blood was not ruled out. The control should have had five chimps inoculated with blood of a healthy donor.[111]

In other words, it's possible that the elevated levels in the 1978 study came about simply because of the experimental procedure—that is, the process of injecting blood. Therefore, conclusions should not be drawn. Dr. Köhnlein continues, arguing that the belief in a hepatitis C virus is likely due to the indirect metric of a PCR result:

> At one of the last hepatitis C meetings in Paris, Michael Houghton, one of the co-discoverers of the sequence we now call hepatitis C virus, asked the audience: "Who has ever seen the hepatitis C virus?" Answer: nobody did.
>
> My question: How do we know that a high viral load, which we are measuring with [the] PCR [test], is indeed [an] infectious virus? There is no paper showing a correlation with free infectious virus particles (visible

> with electron microscopy) and a high "viral load." Are we facing a PCR artifact? I am afraid we are.[112]

Dr. Bailey points to additional problematic studies suggesting that the virus hasn't been isolated. As she puts it, "At no stage in history has any scientific publication demonstrated a replication-competent infectious and disease-causing particle that results in hepatitis."[113]

Hepatitis gained notoriety when actress Pamela Anderson announced in 2002 that she had contracted the disease and believed she got it after sharing a tattoo needle with her husband, Tommy Lee. However, as Dr. Bailey notes, a toxic lifestyle could easily explain her condition.[114] Anderson announced in 2015 that she had been "cured" of hepatitis C.[115]

Rabies

Rabies refers to a rare but often fatal condition that occurs after being bitten by an animal with the condition. Conventional medical thinking tells us that it's a viral infection.

The CDC reports that in the early 1900s, there were more than a hundred human deaths per year, and since the 1960s, the number has dropped to one or two per year.[116] Like chicken pox, the death figures are tiny. But because rabies is a significant part of the lore about viruses, it bears mention.

One of Christine Massey's Freedom of Information requests submitted to the CDC in 2021 asked for records of purifying the rabies virus. She received a response from the Poxvirus and Rabies branch of the CDC, which explicitly said that their procedure does not involve purification prior to the typical cell-culture procedure.[117] Thus, the existence of a rabies virus hasn't been established. It follows, then, that something that hasn't been conclusively shown to exist can't be shown to be transmissible and disease-causing.

However, rabies has a special place in the history of virology because of Louis Pasteur's work. He famously developed a rabies vaccine in the late 19th century. But what isn't often discussed is the barbaric method he employed to make it. He injected pieces of the spinal cord of a dog (believed to have died from rabies) into the brain of a rabbit, and repeated this process by passing spinal cord material, via brain injection, from rabbit to rabbit. Immunologist Rino Rappuoli notes that Pasteur "[passed] it from rabbit to rabbit 20–25 times." Pasteur then dehydrated the spinal cord material from the last dead rabbit in the chain for use in his vaccine.[118]

The Pasteur vaccine is said to have cured a young boy named Joseph Meister in 1885 after he was bitten by a dog believed to have had rabies. Pasteur had never isolated a rabies virus,[119] nor did the technology exist at that time to be able to see a virus. The virus was just assumed to be there. Physician/surgeon Millicent Morden noted, "Medicine has heard much of the startling cure of Joseph Meister by Pasteur. Little mention is made of the fact that three relatives of the Meister boy were bitten by the same dog, and without benefit of the Pasteur treatment, recovered completely."[120]

Additionally, historian Gerald Geison—who studied Pasteur's private notebooks and wrote a book about it published in 1995 by Princeton University Press—mentions that Meister was asymptomatic. He had been bitten, but it was unclear if he would come down with the fatal condition.[121] Therefore, it is unclear whether the vaccine is what allowed the boy to live. As Geison put it, the boy had "an indeterminate chance of surviving without [the vaccine]."[122] In spite of this, the vaccine was lauded as a savior, Pasteur's status as a hero was cemented, and there has since been a persistent belief that rabies is a virus cured by a vaccine designed to counteract the virus.

Dr. Morden added the following (as published in Dr. Eleanor McBean's 1957 book *The Poisoned Needle*): "There are over 3,000 deaths on record in reports from the Pasteur Institute of people bitten by dogs. All died after treatments. On the other hand, the record of the London Hospital, a few years ago, showed 2,668 persons bitten by angry dogs; not one of them developed [rabies symptoms], and not one had been treated by the Pasteur method."[123]

In the United States, mass vaccination of dogs began in 1947.[124] According to the CDC's data, the number of human rabies cases was already low before the vaccine was introduced (no more than roughly fifty cases in the country per year). Human cases were on the decline prior to the vaccine's introduction and continued to decline significantly after the vaccine rollout. The number of cases has been less than ten per year for decades. To the extent that the CDC's data can be trusted on rabies cases in domestic animals, the animal cases were up and down prior to mass vaccination. In the immediate years prior to mass animal vaccination, cases were dropping, but they significantly dropped after the vaccine was introduced.

Whether the vaccine *caused* these declines is an open debate. Determining causation always requires looking at a multitude of other factors, not just a correlation.

For example, it's difficult to know if symptoms were recategorized or labeled as another disease (which is what seems to have happened with polio, and perhaps even with chicken pox). Diseases such as canine distemper, encephalitis, and other neurological conditions bear some resemblance to symptoms of rabies. Any such categorization problems would be a complicating factor when analyzing the data and evaluating the alleged efficacy of the vaccine.[125]

Interestingly, alleged rabies-like viruses exist that don't carry the same stigma that rabies has, such as: Lagos bat virus, Mokola virus, Duvenhage virus, European bat virus 1 and 2, and Australian bat virus. As noted by researcher Mike Stone, "This is a nice, convenient scapegoat, which allows a country to declare itself rabies-free even though the same symptoms of disease still persist."[126]

The more fundamental issue from the No Virus perspective is that the virus hasn't been isolated, so any diagnoses (and associated data)—for both humans and animals—rely on indirect metrics, thereby hindering a complete analysis.

But the big question still lingers: If rabies isn't a virus, what is an alternative hypothesis for this lethal condition? No one knows for sure, but several ideas have been put forward.

Dawn Lester and David Parker note that malnourishment and mistreatment of the animals could play a role. Also, a reported Spanish-flu vaccine side effect was "post-vaccinal encephalitis" (which can cause rabies-like symptoms), so Lester and Parker wonder if the rabies vaccine given to animals might have had a similar side effect.[127] Dr. Samantha Bailey speculates that what's known as rabies could be a poison (more specifically, a neurotoxin) secreted by bacteria within the animal. Under this theory, the toxin would be transferred via trauma (such as a bite)—and there are many examples of other animals that can transfer poisons.[128] In other words, it is not a "virus" or "infection."

Recall Alfred Grafe's explanation of the ancients' view of viruses, in his book *A History of Experimental Virology* (and as mentioned in chapter 2 of this work). The ancient Greeks considered a virus to be a "slimy poison of visible origin. This is illustrated by the dog roaming with rage depicted in Egyptian, Greek and Roman literature."[129] Grafe also noted that the term *ios*, from which the term *virus* emerged, "was the visible poison which caused man and animal alike to become ill or even die. It was recognizable as the venomous secretion of a viper, the poisonous potion from a plant, or the saliva of a rabid dog."[130] Might a "rabid" dog simply refer to a poisoned—and poisonous—dog? That would stand in contrast to the modern view of a virus that regards it specifically as an intracellular parasite.

Black Death

Outbreaks of the plague have been reported in three instances throughout history: the 5th century BCE, the 6th century AD, and the 14th century AD (this one was known as the Black Death). The WHO reports that the case-fatality rate is 30 to 100 percent if left untreated, and more than 50 million people died in Europe due to the Black Death. The WHO states: "Plague is an infectious disease caused by the bacteria *Yersinia pestis*, a zoonotic bacteria, usually found in small mammals and their fleas. It is transmitted between animals through fleas. Humans can be infected through the bite of infected vector fleas; unprotected contact with infectious bodily fluids or contaminated materials; [or] the inhalation of respiratory droplets/small particles from a patient with pneumonic plague."[131]

Dawn Lester and David Parker remark about this narrative: "Nothing could be further from the truth." They note several problems. First, dead rats should have filled the streets, and yet excavations of the cities show little evidence of a massive die-off of rats. Some have postulated that gerbils might have been the primary disease vector instead of rats, but records show no massive die-off of gerbils, either. The disease also traveled faster than can be accounted for by the traditional contagion narrative. And Lester and Parker ask how it could be that fleas would be unaffected if they carried disease-causing bacteria.[132]

A counternarrative is that there were major environmental events that caused "corruption of the air and earth," as speculated by Mike Baillie, a professor at Queen's University in Belfast. His analysis of tree-ring data led him to examine ice-core data, which reveals unusually high levels of ammonium. Baillie comments: "There really is enough information about comets, earthquakes, and ammonium to permit quite serious suggestion that the Black Death was due to an impact by comet debris on 25th January 1348 as witnessed by the major earthquake on that day."[133]

Lester and Parker conclude, "The toxic substances known to be associated with comets and comet debris provide an extremely compelling explanation for the rapid onset of severe respiratory problems, asphyxiation, and death. The medical establishment theory about fleas infected with bacteria that were spread by small animals to humans is entirely unsupported by the evidence."[134]

Summary

Although only a select few diseases have been described in this chapter, the analytical thought process could be applied to any other alleged infectious disease not discussed here. Demonstrating proper isolation of the alleged germ is, of course, an unavoidable prerequisite. Additionally, transmission studies need to be examined with a critical eye—they should have proper controls and ideally would demonstrate transmission in a natural, normal way. Non-germ factors always need to be considered, such as sanitation, toxins, electricity, wireless signals, radiation poisoning, overall lifestyle, nutrition, environmental changes, medications (including vaccines), and many more.

But until rigorous studies are done to investigate these alternative hypotheses, we can't know for sure what is causing illness in various circumstances—which leaves us currently in the realm of speculation. Modern medicine might simply be in a state akin to that of doctors of past generations who didn't realize that scurvy, beriberi, and pellagra were the result of simple nutritional deficiencies.[135] The consensus beliefs *missed* the true cause before. Why couldn't that be happening again in the modern era?

Overall, what's perhaps most striking about this exercise is that there doesn't seem to exist an abundance of quality studies that conclusively demonstrate contagion—let alone studies that approach the level of rigor that one would expect from Koch's or Rivers's postulates. Dr. Thomas Cowan expressed a similar concern following his August 2023 challenge in which he requested from scientists properly designed contagion studies, and yet in return he received studies that were flawed and failed to meet his basic requests. He and his colleagues have been at this since 2020. He says, "[The studies] should be not hard to find. There should be hundreds of these studies. But we can't find them."[136]

CHAPTER 5

VACCINE SAFETY

Vaccines are fundamental to the allopathic model of medicine because germ theory is so central to it. The belief in infectious disease provides the pretext for a "miracle" public-health cure that is said to prevent the spread of germ-based illnesses. Therefore, deconstructing the truth about vaccines is an essential exercise within a critique of allopathic medicine.

In fact, in 2020 the WHO announced its "Immunization Agenda 2030: A Global Strategy to Leave No One Behind." The WHO "envisions a world where everyone, everywhere, at every age, fully benefits from vaccines to improve health and well-being."[1] Is this necessary? From the perspective of terrain theory and the No Virus camp, vaccines don't even make sense.

As discussed in the previous chapter, there are a number of historical examples suggesting that vaccines might *not* have "saved the day," because other factors were actually responsible for declines in disease (such as polio and smallpox). Moreover, Suzanne Humphries, MD; and Roman Bystrianyk, the authors of *Dissolving Illusions* (2013), have aggregated data around many historical illnesses. **They show that by the time vaccines for whooping cough (pertussis), measles, and diphtheria were in widespread use, the death counts associated with each illness had already dropped**

precipitously.[2] What follows are renderings of the graphs shown in their book, which are publicly available at https://dissolvingillusions.com/graphs-images/#Charts.

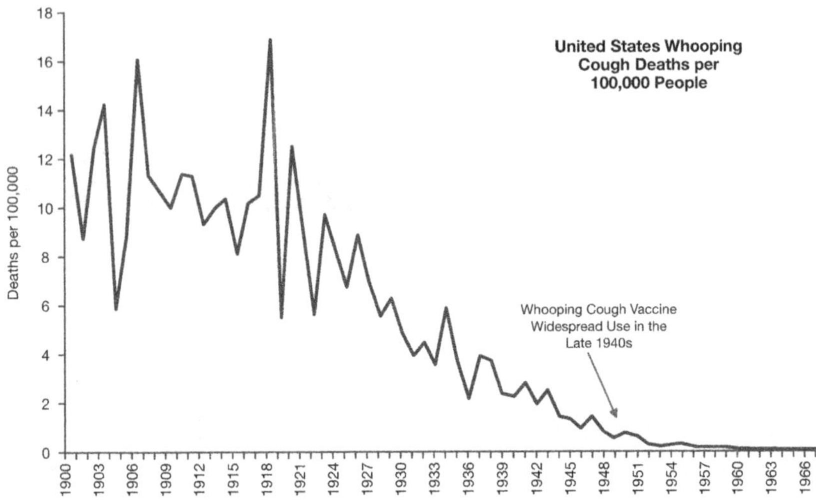

As noted at https://dissolvingillusions.com/graphs-images/#Charts, the graph shows the United States whooping cough mortality rate from 1900 to 1967. (Vital Statistics of the United States 1937, 1938, 1943, 1944, 1949, 1960, 1967, 1976, 1987, 1992; Historical Statistics of the United States—Colonial Times to 1970 Part 1; Health, United States, 2004, US Department of Health and Human Services; Vital Records & Health Data Development Section, Michigan Department of Community Health; US Census Bureau, Statistical Abstract of the United States: 2003; Reported Cases and Deaths from Vaccine Preventable Diseases, United States, 1950–2008.)

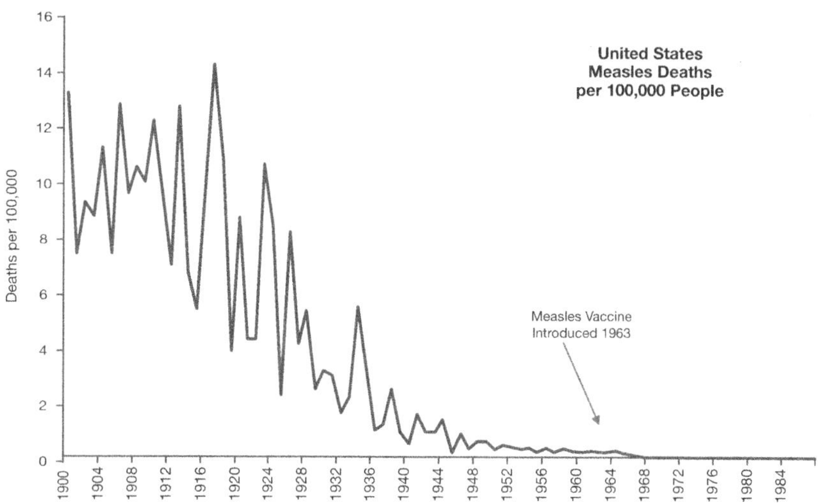

As noted at https://dissolvingillusions.com/graphs-images/#Charts, the graph shows the United States measles mortality rate from 1900 to 1987. (Vital Statistics of the United States 1937, 1938, 1943, 1944, 1949, 1960, 1967, 1976, 1987, 1992; Historical Statistics of the United States— Colonial Times to 1970 Part 1; Health, United States, 2004, US Department of Health and Human Services; Vital Records & Health Data Development Section, Michigan Department of Community Health; US Census Bureau, Statistical Abstract of the United States: 2003; Reported Cases and Deaths from Vaccine Preventable Diseases, United States, 1950–2008.)

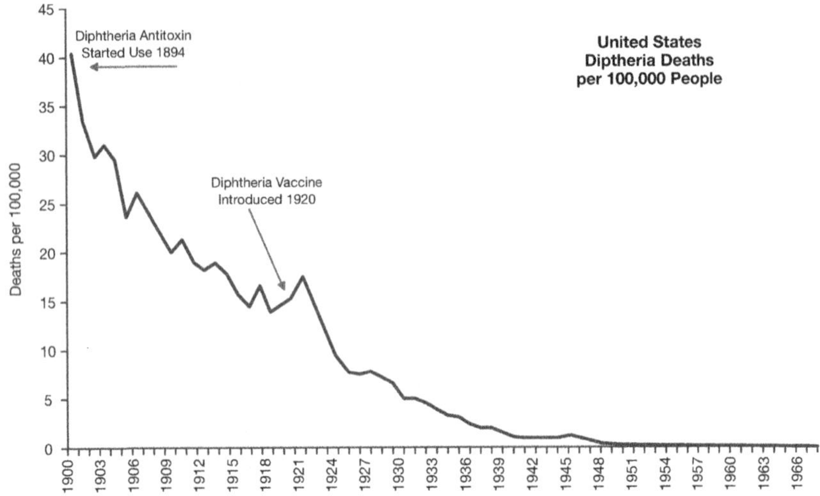

As noted at https://dissolvingillusions.com/graphs-images/#Charts, the graph shows the United States diphtheria mortality rate from 1900 to 1967. (Vital Statistics of the United States 1937, 1938, 1943, 1944, 1949, 1960, 1967, 1976, 1987, 1992; Historical Statistics of the United States— Colonial Times to 1970 Part 1; Health, United States, 2004, US Department of Health and Human Services; Vital Records & Health Data Development Section, Michigan Department of Community Health; US Census Bureau, Statistical Abstract of the United States: 2003; Reported Cases and Deaths from Vaccine Preventable Diseases, United States, 1950–2008.)

Similarly, diseases sometimes subside on their own. In the second half of the 19th century, there were significant drops in mortality for certain conditions *without* vaccines: typhoid (80 percent mortality drop), scarlet fever (80 percent mortality drop), tuberculosis (50 percent mortality drop), and the bowel diseases dysentery and cholera (30 percent mortality drop).[3]

But beyond questions of efficacy, vaccine safety is an essential consideration in the quest to understand disease in the modern world. Vaccines undoubtedly contain ingredients that are known to be toxic (more on this to come). Therefore, it's important to examine the extent to which vaccines are quietly contributing to disease rather than preventing it.

Obstacles to Challenging the Narrative

Science is supposed to be a process that encourages criticism, yet the science of vaccines isn't supposed to be questioned. This became clear to much of the world during the COVID-19 era, in which many people expressed concerns over rushed vaccines that had received no long-term testing. One political poll published in January 2022 even showed that nearly 50 percent of US Democrat voters believed that governments "should be able to fine or imprison individuals who publicly question the efficacy of the existing COVID-19 vaccines on social media, television, radio, or in online or digital publications."[4]

Along these lines, censorship has been rampant under the guise of preventing the spread of "misinformation"—a vague term that in practice shuts down the ability to question prevailing narratives. In February 2021, CBS reported that Facebook had taken "more aggressive steps to combat conspiracy theories and misinformation about vaccines."[5] Similarly, in September 2021, NPR published an article titled "YouTube Is Banning All Content That Spreads Misinformation."[6]

Measures such as this have likely been influenced by government officials. The *Washington Post* reported in September 2023 that judges in the U.S. Court of Appeals for the 5th circuit "found that pressure from the White House and the CDC affected how social media platforms handled posts about COVID-19 in 2021, as the Biden administration sought to encourage the public to obtain vaccinations."[7]

Additionally, the government's own FDA had been explicitly attempting to conceal information about Pfizer's COVID-19 vaccine…*for seventy-five years.* An analysis of Pfizer's documents is available at https://dailyclout.io/. Select reports and a summary analysis were released in a December 2022 compendium titled *Pfizer Document Analysis Report* (published by War Room and DailyClout). The summary states:

> **The Food and Drug Administration (FDA) asked a federal court to allow them 75 years to publicly release Pfizer's COVID-19 vaccine data submitted to the agency. The court ordered the FDA to immediately begin releasing 55,000 pages of the Pfizer vaccine data per month into the public domain.** This report draws from the original analysis of the War Room/DailyClout team of over 3,000 expert volunteers who analyzed the documents released to date, including: Pfizer's COVID-19 vaccine clinical trial data [and] Pfizer's real-world data during the first 12 weeks of its COVID-19 vaccine roll-out from December 1, 2020, through February 28, 2021.[8] [emphasis added]

The analysis of Pfizer's previously hidden documents provided significant revelations, a brief synopsis of which is given by War Room and DailyClout:

> Pfizer's claim of 95% efficacy was based on only a tiny number of COVID-19 cases in the clinical trials—170 cases in over 40,000 trial participants. A measure of vaccine efficacy among such a small sample of COVID-19 cases is too insignificant to generalize to hundreds of millions of people in the population....
>
> Contrary to public statements by Pfizer and FDA, both were aware of data showing that the vaccine ingredients travel from the injection site through the bloodstream, [and] cross important blood-organ barriers (including at the brain, testes, and ovaries)....
>
> Pfizer did not expect more than 158,000 separate adverse events to be reported during the initial 12-week rollout and had to hire a small army of 2,400 additional, full-time staff to manage the case load. Despite these additional staff, Pfizer could not determine the outcome in over 20,000 people reporting vaccine injuries....
>
> As Pfizer tracked adverse events during the first 12 weeks of the vaccine rollout, 270 pregnant women

> reported a vaccine injury, but Pfizer only followed 32 of them and 28 of their babies died. This is a shocking 87.5% fetal death rate....
>
> Pfizer did not evaluate vaccine adverse effects on male fertility during clinical trials because the company was in a rush, stating that the absence of reproductive toxicity data was necessary to speed its vaccine development and meet the allegedly urgent health need. Yet Pfizer's trial documents show that the company knew its vaccine ingredients (the lipid nanoparticles)...pass the blood-testicular barrier and that previous studies had shown that nanoparticles accumulate in the testes and cause reproductive harm by adversely affecting sperm quality, quantity, morphology, and motility.[9]

This information is a far cry from the constant messaging that says the vaccine is "safe and effective." There has been an obvious concealment of information—for those willing to engage with sources outside of the "mainstream." And yet those who simply ask scientific questions are often derided as "antivaxxers."

Things weren't always so extreme, however. In the 2022 book *Turtles All the Way Down: Vaccine Science and Myth,* edited by members of Robert F. Kennedy Jr.'s Children's Health Defense (but written anonymously), the authors show that asking *some* questions used to be more permissible:

> In 1976, the CBS network's famed *60 Minutes* show aired its prime-time investigation on the fabricated "swine flu" epidemic. Only one person had died of the flu, while millions received a rushed vaccine, which was later withdrawn. More than 450 vaccinated people developed paralyzing Guillain-Barré syndrome, and at least 25 died. In 1982, NBC aired *DPT: Vaccine Roulette,* an hour-long documentary on children who had been hurt by the DPT (diphtheria, pertussis, tetanus) vaccine, produced by journalist Lea Thompson. This type of program, which created a public outcry at the time, is unfortunately no longer allowed on US television. The

last person to attempt injecting some vaccine truth was talk-show host Katie Couric, who in 2013 interviewed a mother whose daughter died shortly after receiving the HPV vaccine, Gardasil. Following the airing of the show, Couric was immediately attacked by every major news outlet for, in her own words, "[spending] too much time on the serious adverse events that have been reported in very rare cases following the vaccine." She was quick to issue a public apology, thus, presumably, paying the price for her "dire mistake" and saving her career. To date, no one in mainstream media has dared to follow in her footsteps.

Thus, when even the voice of the injured was no longer allowed to be heard, media reporting of vaccine-related issues became completely one-sided: Only vociferous proponents of vaccines are now allowed to speak—as the ordained priests of "Science."[10]

The Childhood-Vaccine Schedule

Of particular concern in an exploration of vaccine safety is the increasing number of vaccines given to children. If it can be demonstrated that vaccines carry health dangers, then the society-wide impact of childhood vaccination is of great importance. That is, children could be destined to a life of health issues, only to then be managed by the dominant allopathic system. That would be a good thing financially for the pharmaceutical industry because it would mean a constant stream of customers—not only in terms of the vaccines themselves, but also in terms of medications taken later in life to treat long-term conditions arising from the vaccines.

Childhood vaccines have become a growing concern in the US since the passage of The National Childhood Vaccine Injury Act in 1986. **This gave vaccine manufacturers effective immunity from liability.** They needed that liability protection because of the lawsuits they were facing.[11] The act states: "No person may bring a civil action for damages in the amount greater than $1,000 or in an unspecified amount against a vaccine administrator or manufacturer in a State or Federal court for damages arising from a vaccine-related injury or death."[12] This effectively eliminates any financial incentive to make vaccines safe—because the manufacturers are protected. On the other hand, it increases the incentive to create and sell more vaccines.

And that's precisely what has happened since 1986. The number of vaccines for children in the United States has dramatically increased. In 1962, the childhood vaccine schedule included three vaccine doses; by 1986 the figure had increased to twenty-five doses; and as of 2023—after the vaccine makers had secured liability protection in 1986—the number of doses has skyrocketed to at least seventy-three. **Twenty-eight of those doses come in a child's first year.**[13]

What follows is an illustration of these changes over time, re-created from *Vax-Unvax* (2023) by Robert F. Kennedy Jr. and Brian Hooker, PhD.

Year	Vaccine Doses (U.S. Childhood Schedule)
1962 (3 doses)	OVP; Smallpox; DTP
1986 (25 doses)	DTP (2 months); OVP (2 months); DTP (4 months); OVP (4 months); DTP (6 months); MMR (15 months); DTP (18 months); OVP (18 months); HIB (2 years); DTP (4 years); OVP (4 years); Td (15 years)
2023 (73 doses)	Hep B (birth); Hep B (2 months); Rotavirus (2 months); DTaP (2 months); HIB (2 months); PCV (2 months); IPV (2 months); Rotavirus (4 months); DTaP (4 months); HIB (4 months); PCV (4 months); IPV (4 months); DTaP (6 months); HIB (6 months); Hep B (6 months); PCV (6 months); IPV (6 months); COVID-19* (6 months); Influenza (6 months); Rotavirus (6 months); COVID-19* (7 months); Influenza (7 months); HIB (12 months); Influenza (12 months);

Year	Vaccine Doses (U.S. Childhood Schedule)
2023 (73 doses), continued	MMR (12 months); PCV (12 months); Varicella (12 months); Hep A (12 months); DTaP (18 months); Hep A (18 months); Influenza (24 months); Influenza (3 years); DTaP (4 years); IPV (4 years); Influenza (4 years); MMR (4 years); Varicella (4 years); Influenza (5 years); Influenza (6 years); Influenza (7 years); Influenza (8 years); Influenza (9 years); HPV (9 years); Influenza (10 years); HPV (10 years); Influenza (11 years); HPV (11 years); Tdap (12 years); Influenza (12 years); Meningococcal (12 years); Influenza (13 years); Influenza (14 years); Influenza (15 years); Influenza (16 years); Meningococcal (16 years); Influenza (17 years); Influenza (18 years)

Re-created from page 2 of *Vax-Unvax* (2023) by Robert F. Kennedy Jr. and Brian Hooker, PhD. Per the authors' note: "Doses are calculated based on DTaP/Tdap counting as 3 doses and MMR counting as 3 doses (as each are trivalent vaccines). The rest of the schedule is single valent. There are 6 DTaP/Tdaps on the schedule for a total of 18 doses. There are two MMRs on the schedule for a total of 6 doses. There are 49 remaining single-valent for a total of 49+18+6=73 doses. *COVID-19 [refers to] primary series only."

While vaccine makers are effectively immune from liability, there *is* a way to receive compensation for vaccine injuries. It's through a "Vaccine Court," heard by the U.S. Court of Federal Claims, in which the HHS is the respondent—with the support of the Department of Justice. The vaccine maker is not the defendant.[14] (Note: The HHS finds itself in the curious position of defending against claims of vaccine injuries while also being responsible for ensuring vaccine safety.[15])

As of September 2023, this court has had to pay out roughly $5 billion due to vaccine injuries since 1988.[16] But $5 billion appears to be too low. A study conducted from 2007 to 2010 by Harvard Pilgrim Health Care found the following: **"Adverse events from drugs and vaccines are common, but underreported....Fewer than 1 percent of vaccine adverse events are reported."[17] That implies that there could be more than *$500 billion* in vaccine injury damages if all injuries were reported and brought to court.** [emphasis added]

Why are there so many unreported vaccine injuries? The Harvard Pilgram Healthcare study found: "Barriers to reporting include a lack of clinician awareness, uncertainty about when and what to report, as well as the burdens of reporting: reporting is not part of clinicians' usual workflow, takes time, and is duplicative."[18] Furthermore, if there are long-term side effects from a vaccine, it can be difficult to trace with certainty whether they came from the vaccine. Thus, many of these long-term cases are likely lost.

Vaccine Ingredients

The CDC's "Vaccine Excipient Summary" notes that vaccines contain many types of ingredients such as preservatives, adjuvants (designed to "strengthen the immune response"), stabilizers (used "to keep the vaccine potent during transportation and storage"), cell-culture materials, "inactivating" ingredients (used "to kill viruses and inactive toxins"), and antibiotics. The specific ingredients vary by vaccine, but some examples mentioned in the CDC's summary include formaldehyde, thimerosal, aluminum, monosodium glutamate (MSG), FD&C Yellow #6 aluminum lake dye, polysorbate 80, bovine serum albumin, Madin Darby Canine Kidney (MDCK) cell protein, egg protein, chicken protein, processed bovine gelatin, and a long list of others.[19]

Some vaccines also contain cells from aborted fetuses, as validated by Paul Offit, MD, director of the Vaccine Education Center at the Children's Hospital of Philadelphia. He notes, "One issue, and it tends to be a little contentious, is: Are fetal cells used to make vaccines? The answer is, 'Yes.' There were two elective abortions that were performed in the early 1960s, one in Sweden, one in

England. Those cells that were obtained from those elective abortions have been used to make several vaccines."[20]

The point is that there's a lot of stuff being injected into people, and the ingredients themselves aren't often discussed. It's reasonable to wonder whether injecting these substances has any negative effect on the body, especially babies and young children. Humans *are* exposed to toxins in everyday life, but the mechanism of "delivery" in those natural cases is, for instance, through the skin (via touching); the digestive system (via food); and the lungs (via breathing). In other words, natural intake is not via an injection.

Consider, for instance, formaldehyde—a vaccine ingredient that also appears on the CDC's "Toxic Substances Portal."[21] The National Institutes of Health (NIH) also lists formaldehyde as a known carcinogen.[22] Yet the CDC says on its website that formaldehyde is a "residual inactivating ingredient" in vaccines, and because the amount is so small, "it does not pose a safety concern."[23] The site does not provide a citation or scientific evidence to support this claim.

Thimerosal—a mercury-based preservative—is another ingredient that's gotten a significant amount of attention. Robert F. Kennedy Jr. wrote an entire book about it, published in 2015, titled *Thimerosal: Let the Science Speak, The Evidence Supporting the Immediate Removal of Mercury—a Known Neurotoxin—from Vaccines.*[24]

As of September 2023, the CDC states on its website: "Thimerosal is a mercury-based preservative that has been used for decades in the United States in multi-dose vials (vials containing more than one dose) of medicines and vaccines. There is no evidence of harm caused by the low doses of thimerosal in vaccines, except for minor reactions like redness and swelling at the injection site. However, in July 1999, the Public Health Service agencies, the American Academy of Pediatrics, and vaccine manufacturers agreed that thimerosal should be reduced or eliminated in vaccines as a precautionary measure."[25] One might wonder why such precautionary measures needed to be taken if it were true that "there is no evidence of harm" except "minor reactions." The fact that they took precautions seems to be an admission that the substance is dangerous.

Aluminum is another often-discussed vaccine ingredient. The CDC lists nearly thirty vaccines that include aluminum. Dr. Samantha Bailey comments, "When I was training as a doctor, we weren't given much information about aluminum. With regard to its being an adjuvant in vaccines, it was barely glossed over. We were mostly instructed to watch for aluminum toxicity in chronic kidney failure in people on hemodialysis....They teach doctors almost exclusively about *acute* aluminum toxicity, which is almost never seen, while ignoring *chronic* toxicity—because it could result in major problems for major industries, including Big Pharma."[26]

The CDC says: "Aluminum salts, such as aluminum hydroxide, aluminum phosphate, and aluminum potassium sulfate have been used safely in vaccines for more than 70 years."[27]

The Informed Consent Action Network filed a Freedom of Information Act request in 2019, asking for human or animal studies establishing the safety of injecting infants and children with aluminum.[28] The NIH responded several months later, stating that "**no records responsive to your request were located.**" Their letter mentions all of the organizations that searched their files, including: the NIH Office of Intramural Research, the National Institute of Allergies and Infectious Diseases, and the Eunice Kennedy Shriver National Institute of Child Health and Human Development.[29] And yet not a single study was cited. [emphasis added]

Aluminum is a known toxin. Qiao Niu remarks in a 2018 article in *Advances in Experimental Medicine and Biology*: "Aluminum can affect our health, [and] especially impair [the] central nervous system. The important damage is cognitive impairment in aluminum-exposed peoples [*sic*], Alzheimer's disease and other neurodegenerative disorders have been related with aluminum exposure, and aluminum has been proposed as etiology."[30]

Furthermore, Christopher Exley, a professor of bioinorganic chemistry at Keele University in the United Kingdom, talks about aluminum in vaccines more specifically. His paper, titled

"The toxicity of aluminum in humans," published in *Morphologie* in 2016, states:

> Human exposure to aluminum is inevitable and, perhaps, inestimable....Biologically reactive aluminum is present throughout the human body and while, rarely, it can be acutely toxic, much less is understood about chronic aluminum toxicity....
>
> An argument, which is often brought out with respect to the putative toxicity of aluminum in vaccines, is that the amount of aluminum injected is insignificant with respect to human exposure by other routes. However, this thinking does not account for what we now know unequivocally, which is that significant amounts of aluminum adjuvant can be collected from injection sites and transported throughout the body and delivered in potentially acute amounts to target sites which would normally only receive or be subjected to very low but persistent exposure to aluminum. Recent evidence not only points towards the cellular trafficking of aluminum away from the injection site but also its potential delivery to the brain. **Imagine the potential catastrophic consequences of such for an infant receiving multiple vaccinations containing aluminum adjuvants during the first few months of life.**[31] [emphasis added]

Vaccine Safety Testing

Given the range of ingredients in vaccines, a natural question arises: How exactly is safety being established? In *Turtles All the Way Down*, the authors note that the vast majority of physicians and researchers are completely unaware of the manner in which vaccine safety trials are designed and conducted."[32] **The surprising truth is that virtually no childhood vaccines are tested against a proper control group. A proper control group would be given an inert placebo, such as salt water, instead of a vaccine.**

Consider a crude, hypothetical example: Let's say a study wanted to determine whether people get sick if they accidentally consume a new rat poison, developed by Chemical Company A. Researchers could conduct a study in which they give one group of people the rat poison and others in the study water. Those who receive water would be the group that received the "placebo." Researchers would then monitor the adverse health events that occur in participants from both groups. They'd likely find that the people who consumed the rat poison got sick much more often.

But what if the researchers decided to do a different version of the study? Instead of giving the second group water, they give them the rat poison made by Chemical Company B. Perhaps the results would show that the people who took Chemical Company A's rat poison had roughly the same number of adverse health events as the group that took Chemical Company B's rat poison. The researchers could then conclude that Chemical Company A's rat poison is roughly as safe as Chemical Company B's.

This is similar to the way in which childhood-vaccine safety trials are run. Researchers test the safety of one vaccine against what they *call* a "placebo"—but it's not really a placebo. Their placebo is another vaccine, such as an older generation of the vaccine. **The placebo isn't an inert solution like salt water.** So the *relative* safety of one vaccine versus another is being tested—not the absolute safety of the vaccine versus an inert placebo. Attorney Aaron Siri even created a publicly available list of problematic vaccine studies in an August 2023 article called "Proof Regarding the Clinical Trials Relied Upon by the FDA to License the Childhood Vaccines on the CDC Childhood Vaccine Schedule."[33]

In *Turtles All the Way Down*, the authors also walk through the details for certain childhood vaccines, such as the DTaP vaccine (Diphtheria-Tetanus-acellular-Pertussis). The short version, in their words, is: "The safety of GlaxoSmithKline's 5-in-1 and 4-in-1 vaccine was tested against the triple vaccine (DTaP), which was tested against the older-generation vaccine (DTP), whose safety was never tested in a [randomized-controlled trial] with a placebo control group."[34] It's a house of cards.

Some experts, such as Dr. Offit, have openly defended the methodology, arguing that it would be unethical to give participants an inert placebo rather than a potentially lifesaving vaccine.[35] This, of course, presupposes that the vaccines are safe and effective when in fact the point of scientific studies is to determine whether that's true. One could argue the reverse—that it's unethical *not* to use true placebos, because without them, the dangers of vaccines can't be determined properly.[36] In the FDA approval process for many other drugs, pharmaceutical companies *do* use true placebos.[37]

Another consideration is that the childhood-vaccine schedule entails receiving many vaccines in a short amount of time. That means placebo-controlled safety studies should be run to test the effects of taking multiple vaccines in a short period—not just studying the effects of taking one vaccine at a time. Though tedious, if scientists wanted to be *really* thorough, they'd run studies on injections of each vaccine ingredient—one by one—versus the injection of an inert placebo. That might help identify whether particular ingredients are dangerous. Studies conducted on full vaccines simply examine the effect of a mixed fluid without looking at the individual components.

Vaccine studies are also notoriously short in duration, so researchers might miss patterns of long-term health problems that could be associated with the vaccines. **Dr. Anthony Fauci echoed this sentiment in 1999, arguing that if agencies rush to approve vaccines, "then you find out that it takes twelve years for all hell to break loose; then what would you have done?"[38]**

Kennedy and his coauthor, Brian Hooker, PhD, add in their book *Vax-Unvax* (2023): "Despite Dr. Fauci's warning, FDA clinical safety studies generally last for a relatively short duration, precluding the detection of long-term health effects. For example, researchers monitored vaccine recipients in the Engerix-B (hepatitis B) trial for adverse events for only four days after injection. Similarly, researchers monitored vaccine recipients in the Infantrix (DTaP) clinical trial for adverse events for only four days after injection. For the ActHIB (Haemophilus influenzae B), scientists monitored patients for a mere forty-eight hours after injection. That's it!"[39]

Del Bigtree, host of *The Highwire*, recalls that in May 2017, he and Kennedy were in a meeting with Dr. Francis Collins (the then-head of the NIH) and Dr. Fauci: "[Kennedy]...asked [Fauci] to show us inert placebo-controlled studies for any of the [then] seventy-one recommended vaccine doses. Fauci made a scene of going through a series of file folders that had apparently been rolled in from the NIH archives on a cart. Then, in what appeared to be feigned exasperation, he said none of the studies were there but that he would send them to us. Of course, he never did."[40]

Kennedy then sent a Freedom of Information request to the HHS, asking for copies of long-term, placebo-controlled clinical trials for each childhood vaccine. The HHS admitted in writing that it "did not locate any records" in response to the request.[41]

Furthermore, in 2013, the Institute of Medicine (IOM) reported that "studies designed to examine the longer-term effects of the cumulative number of vaccines or other aspects of the immunization schedule have not been conducted."[42] The report was commissioned by the National Vaccine Program Office of the HHS.

The IOM's 2011 report examined some vaccine adverse events, and for the vast majority they weren't able to determine if the vaccine did or did not cause the health problems. Kennedy and Dr. Hooker write: "Isn't it stunning to comprehend that for almost 90% of the vaccine adverse events [examined, the] CDC has never completed sufficient studies to affirm or rule out a causal relationship? This means it can't know whether these vaccines actually cause harm and certainly can't honestly say that they don't."[43] [emphasis added]

It's a good strategy for health officials, actually. They can claim that there is no evidence for certain adverse events...but they leave out *why* there is no evidence. Maybe there's no evidence because the studies aren't being run. For instance, consider what the ENGERIX-B (hepatitis B) vaccine states in its package insert:

"ENGERIX-B has not been evaluated for carcinogenic or mutagenic potential, or for impairment of male fertility in animals."[44] [emphasis added]

Similarly, it's important to note the lack of long-term data on vaccine *efficacy*. That is, there are basic studies that could help researchers better understand how well a vaccine protects against a given condition—relative to those who don't receive the vaccine. As noted by Dr. Andrew Kaufman: "Vaccine studies don't track a group of children long term and see how many get sick among those who received the vaccine versus those who received the placebo. The basis for getting a vaccine approved is typically whether they show a blood test that's positive for antibodies. The only way to truly determine if the vaccines are effective is to compare vaccinated and unvaccinated groups over a period that's at least over a decade, and likely longer."[45]

Vaxed vs. Unvaxed Studies

Studies of vaccinated people versus unvaccinated people also enable clear comparisons regarding vaccine safety. The intent is not just to look at which groups get sick from the disease that the vaccine is supposed to protect against. Rather, such studies would help determine which group has more heart disease, mental illness, autism, cancer, fertility problems, diabetes, multiple sclerosis, gastrointestinal disorders, asthma, Alzheimer's disease, skin conditions, food allergies, and other health issues.

Kennedy and Dr. Hooker looked at data along these lines. Since the HHS was unable to provide long-term studies in response to Kennedy's request (as mentioned earlier), he then embarked on a research journey with Dr. Hooker to see if there were any studies in the NIH's archive that compared vaccinated to unvaccinated populations. Del Bigtree recalls, "Slowly, they began finding studies that either deliberately or inadvertently made these comparisons. Over the next year, [Kennedy and Dr. Hooker] published these studies one at a time on [Kennedy's] Instagram and on the Children's Health Defense's website....Then, in February 2021, Instagram evicted [Kennedy] from its platform."[46] Two and a half years later, in August 2023, Kennedy and Dr. Hooker published the results in their book *Vax-Unvax: Let the Science Speak*.

The studies show, over and over, that unvaccinated populations have fewer health problems than vaccinated ones. Kennedy and Dr. Hooker aggregated more than one hundred peer-reviewed articles. **One cluster of those studies shows that compared to unvaccinated groups, vaccinated groups have more ADD and/or ADHD; allergies; asthma; autism; developmental disabilities, learning disabilities, or neurodevelopmental disorders; eczema; ear infections; gastrointestinal disorders; respiratory infections; and seizures.**[47]

The Sacred Cow

There are many "anomalies" that seem to contradict the dictum that "vaccines are safe and effective." One might wonder why more progress hasn't been made toward resolving the debates that persist. The stakes are very high given how many injections are being given to children and how much pressure was placed on the global population to take the COVID-19 vaccine.

Vaccines have served as a mechanism by which the population can be controlled. During the COVID-19 era, the messaging was essentially: "If you want to have normal participation in society, you must receive as many doses of the vaccine as we tell you, and don't ask questions."

Challenging the sanctity of vaccines is thus an affront to core aspects of the global power structures and to the broader pharmaceutical industry—especially when it's done by credentialed doctors and scientists whom the public might be inclined to listen to. Kennedy and Dr. Hooker elaborate on the way that this dynamic manifests in practice:

> Physicians and scientists who fall out of line with the orthodoxy of vaccinology emerge as heretics and pariahs. The most famous example took place in 1998 when Dr. Andrew Wakefield reported that 8 out of 12 of his

> autistic patients received the MMR [Measles, Mumps, and Rubella] vaccine prior to developing gastrointestinal symptoms and recommended further study. The level of fallout was epic. Dr. Wakefield lost his medical license, reputation, and country over this brief statement he made in a now-retracted 1998 paper in the medical journal *Lancet.* So far-reaching was his persecution that the term "Wakefielded" is now used to describe the systematic gaslighting and vilification of physicians and scientists who dare to challenge vaccine orthodoxies by the government, media, and pharmaceutical enterprises. Since 1998, many other medical practitioners have paid dearly for researching vaccine risks and giving patients options that deviate from the CDC schedule. Scientists pursuing honest vaccine safety research have their peer-reviewed studies retracted and pulled out of circulation under dubious circumstances. Many have lost careers, revenue, and reputation as scientific and medical communities, government agencies, and media marginalize and condemn them.[48]

In spite of these obstacles, there seems to be increasing momentum toward getting to the bottom of the vaccine debate. And that's a positive development in the movement to transcend the allopathic model of medicine.

PART II
WHY IS CONSCIOUSNESS RELEVANT TO MEDICINE?

CHAPTER 6

PHYSICALISM VS. IDEALISM

So far, many problematic aspects of the allopathic model have been discussed, but now comes perhaps its biggest flaw: allopathic medicine is nowhere close to understanding what a human being is—and that's because its view about the nature of reality itself is deeply flawed. In this chapter, I explore fundamental aspects of what allopathic medicine is missing, which will lead to a discussion in the next chapter about the vast implications for health and disease.

The Nature of Reality—Opposing Views

The mainstream scientific paradigm, and that of allopathic medicine, views humans to be physical beings made of atoms: The human body emerged through a random evolutionary process since an event started the universe, theorized to have been the "Big Bang," roughly 13.8 billion years ago. After the universe began, atoms started colliding and engaging in chemical reactions, until, randomly, self-replicating molecules formed, which then led to the evolution of the human species (among others). Humans developed brains, and through that structure they were able to have a subjective inner awareness—a sense of experiencing life—commonly known as *consciousness.*

The human body has a finite period during which it functions, and then it shuts down and dies. At that point, the body's consciousness ceases as well. Furthermore, under this model, humans exist within a universe that is fundamentally random and meaningless. Human life has no more meaning than what one arbitrarily decides. That is, there isn't any meaning built into the fabric of reality. Ultimately, the human is just a biological robot.

This perspective reduces all of life to *the physical.* It is a metaphysical perspective sometimes known as *physicalism* or *scientific materialism* (frequently leading to atheism or agnosticism). This view can be regarded as the mainstream scientific *meta*paradigm for thinking about the nature of reality itself; it is the paradigm on which all other paradigms are based. Therefore, it is the fundamental presupposition used to evaluate life, including the human body and the treatment thereof (that is, medicine).

But for many reasons, physicalism is an inappropriate presupposition about the nature of reality.

From a philosophical perspective, physicalism *lacks parsimony*—meaning that it invokes more assumptions than are needed to explain reality adequately. It presupposes a reality that existed before all forms of consciousness, and says consciousness came later, after a long evolutionary process derived from inert matter.

Why is this problematic? It's because of something very basic: consciousness is required in order to experience anything. And yet physicalism postulates that the universe existed before anything was able to experience it. That *could* theoretically be true, but it is inherently unverifiable. If there wasn't any consciousness when the universe began, then there isn't a direct way to validate its existence. Only indirect inferences can be made.[1]

On the contrary, consciousness (similarly referred to as *mind*) is something that can be readily verified by everyone at this moment. It is within mind that we are even able to ask such questions about the nature of reality and medicine. Physicalism's belief in the existence of matter outside of consciousness, on the other hand, is unknowable and unverifiable. **As Bernardo Kastrup, PhD, puts**

it, "We do *not*—and fundamentally *cannot*—know matter as confidently as we know mind."[2] From the perspective of Occam's Razor—"the simplest solution is usually the best"—physicalism is therefore inferior to a consciousness-centric metaphysics. [emphasis added]

Such an alternative to physicalism is known as *idealism*, which posits that all reality is made of mind. This is, in fact, our experiential reality: everything that one sees, feels, hears, smells, and touches is a sensation arising *within* one's own consciousness. We interpret a physical world "out there" through our sensory organs, but in reality, everything ever experienced is a "modulation" of one's own consciousness (to use philosopher Rupert Spira's terminology). As Dr. Kastrup says, "We have come to automatically *interpret* the felt concreteness of the world as evidence that the world is outside consciousness. But this is an unexamined artifact of subliminal thought-models. Our only access to the world is through sense perception....The notion that there is a world outside and independent of [experience] is an *explanatory model*, not an empirical fact."[3]

A more parsimonious way of looking at reality is to start with consciousness as the basis of reality itself. In other words, what we call the "physical world" is simply the product of a single, primordial consciousness, of which each of our individual minds is a part. Dr. Kastrup likens all of reality to a stream of consciousness in which each of us is an individual whirlpool.[4]

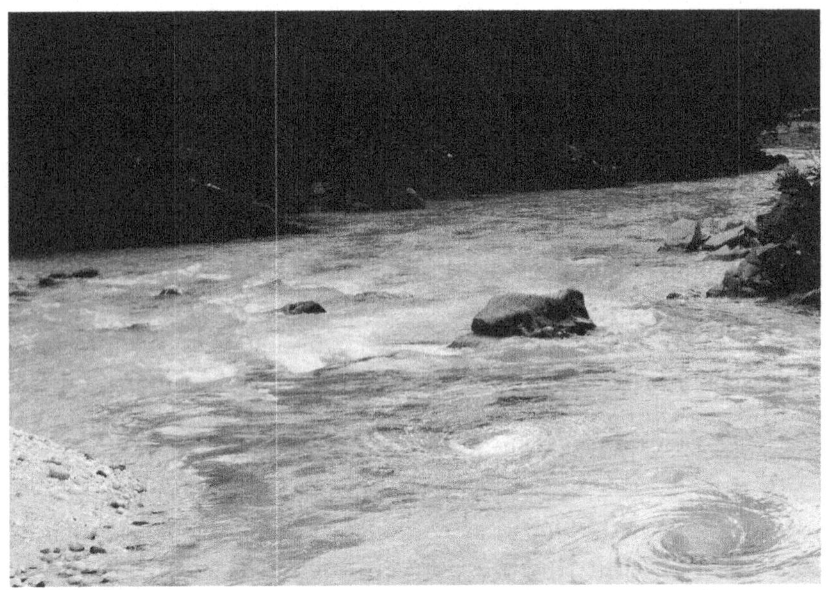

The visual shown above is an illustration of Dr. Bernardo Kastrup's metaphor. He compares consciousness to an infinite stream of water. Each of us is an individuated whirlpool within the stream, and yet at the same time we are fundamentally interconnected because we are part of the same stream. Each whirlpool is thus akin to an individual mind, which is part of the broader, overarching mind. For more on this metaphor, see Dr. Kastrup's book titled *Why Materialism Is Baloney*.

The underlying consciousness—which serves as the substrate for all existence—has *dissociative identity disorder* in the form of individuated minds with which each of us identifies.[5] Consciousness also exists beyond our perceptions of space and time.

This perspective aligns with the conclusions of ancient traditions and resembles what many people have reported when they have spiritually transformative experiences (such as near-death states, psychedelic accounts, meditation experiences, and so on). Additionally, early quantum physicists, such as Nobel Prize winner Max Planck, echoed these sentiments about consciousness versus matter. He stated in 1931, "I regard consciousness as fundamental. I regard matter as derivative from consciousness."[6] Similarly, Nobel Prize winner Erwin Schrödinger said, "In truth, there is only One Mind."[7]

Thus, idealism implies that the body is an individuated vessel or vehicle of consciousness rather than the producer of consciousness. It's a complete flip. As such, "the soul" is an individuated sliver of consciousness that inhabits a body.

The diagram that follows, adapted from the work of Dean Radin, PhD,[8] and used in my other books, illustrates the perspective of idealism, which can be called the "One Mind," for short. The One Mind itself could be likened to what some call "God." The figure shown is a mere two-dimensional approximation of something likely much more complex, so it should not be regarded as a precise metaphysical rendition.

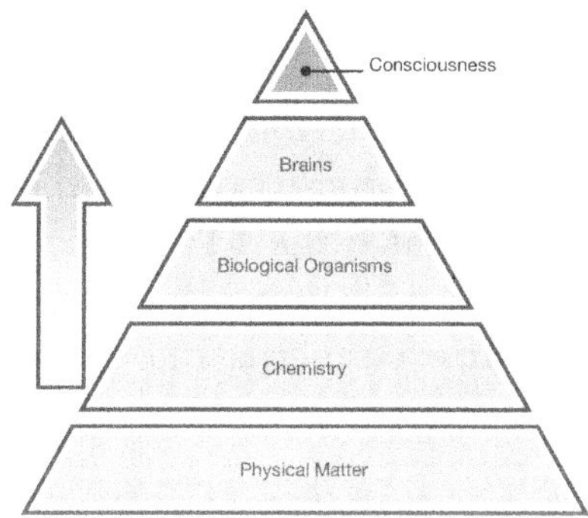

Physicalism: The interactions of units of matter (via chemistry) create biological organisms like human beings, which develop brains, out of which consciousness arises. This worldview supports atheism.

Brains
Biological Organisms
Chemistry
Physical Matter
Consciousness

The "One Mind" view of reality: Consciousness is primary; everything we perceive in the apparently material world is simply a modulation of consciousness itself.[9] This perspective supports a spiritual worldview found at the core of many religious traditions.

The Hard Problem of Consciousness

One of physicalism's big problems is its inability to explain where consciousness comes from. Philosophers and neuroscientists even call it the "hard problem" of consciousness (coined by David Chalmers in 1995). The hard problem is essentially that scientists cannot explain how a physical structure like a brain produces nonphysical consciousness. The body is something we can touch; our consciousness isn't.[10]

Scientists have assumed that because the brain is related to conscious experience, the brain must be producing consciousness. Neuroscience has found many neural correlates of consciousness, in fact. For instance, if someone has an accident that damages the part of the brain responsible for vision, the person might have a corresponding change in one's sight. But correlation doesn't necessarily imply causation. Just because firefighters are at a fire doesn't mean that firefighters *caused* the fire.[11]

If the brain/body structure is a *vessel* of consciousness, then perhaps the brain, and other parts of the body, are like antennae that *receive* consciousness. It's like a TV that picks up a signal from outside the set. Damaging the antenna on the television doesn't damage the signal, but it does damage one's ability to watch the TV show on the screen. Therefore, the brain/body structure is important to the way in which we experience life, but our true essence is untouched by what happens to the body.[12]

An analogy can be drawn to driving a certain type of a car: no matter who the driver is, the car has its features and limitations. So the best the driver can do is keep the car well maintained and drive it safely. Analogously, maintaining a clean and healthy bodily vessel allows consciousness to be experienced optimally. That's not how allopathic medicine views the body.

Another way to view the brain/body structure is as a *filter* of consciousness. For instance, this implies that when the brain's functioning gets "out of the way," a more pure and enriched consciousness can be experienced. There are many phenomena that match this picture. The pattern can be referred to as "less brain, more consciousness."[13]

In near-death experiences (NDEs)—for instance, cases of cardiac arrest and clinical death—upon being resuscitated, people often report that their conscious experience was "realer than real life,"[14] which can include reports of 360-degree vision.[15] Often they report having been immersed in unconditional love, having had otherworldly encounters, or even having received special knowledge. The majority of NDEs are overwhelmingly positive, but a minority are fear-inducing and even hellish. But these miraculous phenomena of consciousness occur at a time when the brain was either barely functioning or completely off. Sometimes NDE survivors were even under general anesthesia at the time of their elaborate experience.[16] The brain was out of the way, and their consciousness was somehow liberated. Less brain, more consciousness—it's almost like a blindfold was lifted. The physicalist model would expect that a lot of brain activity would be needed to have such complex experiences, and yet the opposite occurs.

Similarly, emerging studies on psychedelics show reductions in brain functioning that are associated with an enriched consciousness during a psychedelic trip.[17] Individuals with savant syndrome can have incredible memories, and/or mathematical and musical abilities, and yet have impaired brains. In instances of terminal lucidity, people who've had a brain impairment like Alzheimer's disease snap back into clarity and start speaking normally shortly before dying.[18] As Dr. Kastrup summarizes the situation: "There are certain types of brain function impairment—which under physicalism should correlate with cognitive deficit and under idealism with enriched inner life—that have been shown to be accompanied by enriched inner life. This corroborates idealism and contradicts physicalism."[19] Dr. Kastrup elaborates on such instances in his 2017 *Scientific American* article titled "Transcending the Brain."[20]

Consciousness Anomalies—Psychic Phenomena

There are also many anomalous scientific findings that challenge physicalism. In other words, the findings cannot be well explained by the metaphysics of physicalism, but under idealism (that is, the One Mind) they can be explained easily. For instance, imagine that some of the water from one person's whirlpool gets into another person's whirlpool. That's akin to one person's consciousness slipping into another person's consciousness: in other words, telepathic ability. The One Mind metaphysics is fully compatible with evidence of such psychic phenomena, whereas physicalism views consciousness as something that's stuck inside our skulls. Any "nonlocal" phenomena of consciousness shouldn't happen. So if there exists evidence for *even one* type of nonlocal-consciousness phenomenon, such as psychic ability, then physicalism is again in big trouble.

My book *An End to Upside Down Thinking* (2018) compiles the plethora of scientific evidence for such phenomena, of which a brief portion is summarized here.

Dr. Radin, the chief scientist at the Institute of Noetic Sciences, aggregated some of the key data on nonlocal consciousness in his book *Real Magic* (2018).[21] He shows that there exists strong statistical evidence that the following phenomena are real, based on controlled scientific studies: telepathy (mind-to-mind communication),[22] remote viewing (perceiving something far away, in space and/or time, with the mind alone),[23] precognition (knowing or sensing the future before it happens),[24] and psychokinesis (mind impacting matter without any physical contact).[25] In Dr. Radin's words:

> [Experiments on these phenomena] have exceeded the six-sigma threshold. **This refers to studies where the overall odds against chance, after careful consideration of all known experiments investigating the same topic, are assessed to be over a billion to one.** Each of the experiments used protocols that avoided all known design flaws. An extensive due diligence list of possible design faults has been developed after years of intense scrutiny and criticism of these studies, leading to bulletproof designs.
>
> Each class of experiments has been repeated from a dozen to more than a hundred times by independent investigators at different labs around the world, with each class cumulatively involving hundreds to thousands

> of participants, most of whom were not claiming any special [psychic] abilities.[26] [emphasis added]

For instance, one type of study on telepathy is designed as follows: There are two participants in rooms far away from each other. One of them is shown an image and is asked to mentally "send" what he or she is seeing to the other person. The other person is then shown four images by experimenters and is asked which of the four images was being mentally sent. The person typically guesses correctly roughly 32 percent of the time (plus or minus). If there were no effect at all, the person should guess correctly closer to 25 percent of the time.[27] The several-percentage-point differential seems small, but from a statistical standpoint, it's massive. It's one of those pesky anomalies that physicalism would like to sweep aside.

Furthermore, the US government ran a secret spying program from the 1970s into the 1990s—using "remote viewers" to see things far away, using their mind alone. More than $20 million was invested in the program, and declassified CIA documents explicitly confirm: "Remote viewing is a real phenomenon[;] Implications are revolutionary."[28]

Additionally, Dr. Etzel Cardeña's 2018 paper published in *American Psychologist*—the official peer-reviewed academic journal of the American Psychological Association—provided statistical validation for a variety of psychic phenomena.[29] The fact that such a mainstream journal would publish results like this—in an academic environment that is typically hostile and dismissive toward anything that questions physicalism—is significant.

Statistician Jessica Utts, PhD, the 2016 president of the American Statistical Association, summarizes the accumulated scientific results concisely: **"Using the standards applied to any other area of science, it is concluded that psychic functioning has been well established."**[30] [emphasis added]

Consciousness Anomalies—Surviving Bodily Death

Returning to the whirlpool analogy: If one person's whirlpool delocalizes, the water flows back into the broader stream. Similarly, if a person's body dies, his or her consciousness flows back into the broader "stream" of multidimensional consciousness. By analogy, consciousness never dies; it just transitions into new forms. That's the prediction under the One Mind, whereas under physicalism this is crazy talk.

NDE research supports this, particularly veridical out-of-body experiences.[31] These are instances in which a person claims his or her body was perceiving things from a vantage point outside the body—while the brain was basically dead. Upon being resuscitated, these people's experiences are validated by doctors, family members, or bystanders. In other words, these cases are not mere hallucinations. The implication is that at least some NDEs reflect a functional consciousness without a functional brain. That is, consciousness continues even in the absence of a brain. As stated by NDE researcher and professor emeritus at the University of Virginia Bruce Greyson, MD, "We're left with this paradox that at a time when the brain isn't functioning, the mind is functioning better than ever."[32]

Many recent media accounts of NDEs claim that scientists have invalidated the phenomenon by showing that the brain isn't fully turned off. Therefore, they seem to claim, NDEs come from the brain.

However, no amount of brain activity can explain how someone's consciousness is accurately seeing and hearing things from a vantage point outside his or her body. Additionally, as noted in a 2010 paper by Dr. Greyson, some NDEs include encountering the "spirit" of people not known at the time to have died.[33] That's not explainable by residual brain activity. Furthermore, physicalist scientists have not established that the brain activity they've identified is capable of producing the vast and complex perceptions that people report in NDEs. Finding *some* brain activity is very different from finding brain activity that can explain the elaborate NDE accounts.

In a 2023 paper, cardiologist Dr. Pim van Lommel and Dr. Greyson explain several of the problems with arguments that dismiss NDEs as mere artifacts of brain activity: "Electrical processes do not and cannot explain what enables unconscious patients to see unexpected things in the material world accurately from an out-of-body visual perspective....; to recognize and interact with deceased persons who, in the material world, were not yet known to have died; or to experience greatly enhanced cognition and perception during cardiac arrest or general anesthesia when neuroscientific models deem such complex consciousness to be impossible."[34]

Furthermore, Dr. Greyson writes in his book *After* (2021) that he was part of a multinational team that studied the experiences of people who took any of 165 drugs. They found that the substance ketamine induced states that most closely resembled NDEs. However, there were elements of ketamine experiences that do not appear in NDEs, "which suggests that NDEs are not simply an effect of the drug." Dr. Greyson adds: "The neuroscientist who has most fiercely promoted the ketamine model for NDEs concluded after twelve years of research that he viewed ketamine as 'just another door' to NDEs, and not as actually producing them."[35] Dr. Greyson ultimately found that while various models try to explain away NDEs as a product of something happening in the brain, they ultimately serve as mere analogies because they only capture a "limited feature of NDEs....**None of them adequately describes the entire experience.**"[36] [emphasis added]

There are also instances of "shared-death experiences" in which a healthy person co-lives in the dying process—which is reported to be NDE-like—*with the person who is actually dying*. In other words, it's a healthy person with a normal brain who has the experience. Therefore, these instances are not hallucinations caused by a dying brain...because the person who had the experiences wasn't dying. A paper on this phenomenon, written by William Peters and his colleagues, was published in the peer-reviewed *American Journal of Hospice and Palliative Care* in 2021.[37]

Another category of anomalies comes from alleged communications with the deceased, such as those that occur via psychic "mediums." The Windbridge Research Center has published research using five levels of blinding; and they demonstrate that some mediums accurately know things about dead people, under tightly controlled conditions, which cannot be explained by normal means.[38] The claim here isn't that every person alleging to have psychic abilities is legitimate, but rather that some people sometimes *are* legitimate.

Finally, the University of Virgina's Division of Perceptual Studies has examined more than 2,500 cases of young children who have memories of a life that is not their own. In the strongest cases, researchers link those memories to validated historical records establishing that the alleged person from the "previous life" was in fact a real person. The children are often in the range of two to six years old.[39] (Note: In addition to research conducted by Drs. Ian Stevenson and Jim Tucker at the University of Virginia, also see *Reincarnation as a Scientific Concept: Scholarly Evidence for Past Lives* [2021] by K. S. Rawat and Titus Rivas; and *Signs of Reincarnation: Exploring Beliefs, Cases, and Theory* [2019] by James Matlock.)

Anomalies such as the ones described here pose a major challenge to modern medicine's view of the body.

CHAPTER 7

CONSCIOUSNESS, HEALTH, AND DISEASE

If we accept the One Mind perspective to be an approximation for the nature of reality, rather than physicalism, many new considerations enter the picture. Maybe our minds play a much bigger role in our health than allopathic medicine teaches. In this chapter, I introduce many considerations that the mainstream paradigm misses.[1]

Some of the examples and anecdotes discussed in this chapter require much more scientific analysis before the phenomena can be accepted fully. The intent here is to present a wide range of possibilities that need to be considered in a new paradigm of medicine. That is, the forthcoming examples might stimulate new hypotheses that can be tested scientifically. However, because these areas of research often lack significant funding, there is a corresponding shortage of data.

Mind-Matter Interaction and Healing

One implication of a departure from physicalism, as it relates to medicine, is that the physical world (or what we perceive to be "physical") is actually malleable. That is, the mind can directly influence the world in which we operate.

One of the classic studies, included within the six-sigma-statistical-results group, uses random-number generators. These are machines that generate 1s and 0s in a random fashion, which means that over time there are roughly 50 percent 1s and 50 percent 0s. The basic design is as follows: Experimenters ask people to try to make the machines produce more 1s than 0s, using their minds alone. The results suggest that everyday people are able to do so, but the deviation from chance is small. They're highly statistically significant, however.[2] Some of the experimentation in this domain comes from the Princeton Engineering Anomalies Research Lab that was led by Dr. Robert Jahn, the former dean of Engineering at Princeton University; and his colleagues Brenda Dunne and Roger Nelson, PhD, from 1979 to 2007.[3]

Similarly, Princeton researchers and others have examined the behavior of random-number generators set up all over the world. Most people don't know that they even exist—they're just generating 1s and 0s randomly all day. The researchers look at what happens to the machines' behavior when there is a major global event that is likely to cause a strong, common emotion. They find that the machines behave statistically nonrandomly during many major events.[4] In other words, collective consciousness has a measurable impact on the physical world.

The implications of such phenomena are profound for medicine (and science more broadly). First, people can alter the physical world with the intention of their minds alone. Even if the effect is small, it's not zero. **One might wonder: How is the body then impacted by one's state of mind? What might be the impact of *fear* on the body—an emotion that has been encouraged so heavily by the media and other "authorities" during the COVID-19 era?**

Perhaps the placebo effect is related to this concept. For instance, Shamini Jain, PhD, has aggregated scientific studies on this phenomenon that demonstrate the following: placebos account for

75 percent of the effects of antidepressants, they are instrumental in pain reduction, they can cause changes in the brain, and they can even mimic the efficacy of having real surgery when in fact no surgery was performed.[5]

Similarly, there exists a well-documented "nocebo" effect. It refers to instances in which the *fear* of a negative symptom results in those very symptoms, even when a person is given an inert substance.[6] The implication is that the mind can create symptoms on its own, as long as a negative *expectation* is there. **What does this imply about contagion during a "pandemic"—could people's expectations induce disease and create the *appearance* of contagion?**

A second implication of the random-number-generator studies is that when many people have a strong reaction to a common event, they unknowingly impact the physical world together. Along these lines, in Barry Spivack and Patricia Anne Saunders's book, *An Antidote to Violence* (2020), the authors reference twenty peer-reviewed studies, and more than fifty demonstrations, in which groups of people meditating created markedly peaceful outcomes where there had previously been less peace or disarray (known as the "Maharishi Effect").

One might wonder: Could large groups of people holding the same negative mindset, such as fear, create a negative outcome in the world? Could they induce, or encourage, sickness during "pandemics"? This would be occurring in a seemingly nonlinear and invisible manner, beyond our everyday perceptions.

And even more broadly, what does this mean for science at large? Is it even possible to engage in the scientific method if the variable of "consciousness" cannot be controlled or measured, thereby potentially steering and distorting the results of *all* scientific experiments?

The reality of mind-matter interactions might sound new in the modern era, but it's actually an ancient concept. For example, in the Indian spiritual tradition, enlightened masters are said to develop special powers called *siddhis*, in which they are able to mold reality in significant ways—much more significantly than mere statistical shifts seen in random-number-generator experiments. Dr. Dean

Radin, who studies this from a scientific lens, summarized the powers in his book *Supernormal* (2013). They include the ability to become invisible to others, to levitate, to possess extraordinary strength, and to manipulate "the size, appearance, and condition of the body."[7]

One might then wonder how such concepts could be applied to healing, specifically. In other words, can people use their minds to heal others—particularly through the use of some form of invisible "energy" that science doesn't yet understand? Religious traditions tell many tales of miracle healings, but in the modern era, they're often considered to be fictional accounts because they violate physicalist, allopathic assumptions.

While some studies on so-called energy healing have been conducted in the modern era, one can imagine that the amount of funding that this domain has traditionally received is minuscule compared to areas of allopathic focus (like AIDS, vaccines, and so on). By the same token, because of this dynamic, there are far fewer researchers in this domain—and only a select number of brave scientists are willing to endure the potential backlash from exploring areas traditionally considered to be taboo.

But there are some. One such study was published in 2023 in *Dose Response: An International Journal*. The authors employed a form of energy healing known as the Bengston Healing Method on mice (modeled off of the "hands on" healing work of William Bengston, PhD). The authors preface their findings with important history: "The father of Western medicine, Hippocrates, recognized that certain individuals appear to be able to heal, and described this as 'the force which flows from many people's hands.' A list of the methods used by these purported healers have included laying on of hands, prayer, and induced altered states of consciousness, to name a few."[8]

The authors also summarize the eye-opening results they obtained in the present study: "Previous research on 'healing-with-intent' has reasonably demonstrated the validity of the phenomenon at least when a human healer is present and involved. However, in order for healing to be adopted into more conventional therapies, it must be able to be made scalable. The present study tests the effects of a scalable recording of the Bengston Healing Method [on mice]....**In the breast cancer model, there was significant tumor suppression and a reduction of anemia marker HCT in treated vs control mice.**...While the effects...seem to vary by model, there appears reason to pursue scalable delivery systems."[9] [emphasis added]

Although not every alleged miracle healer is necessarily legitimate, there are indeed some noteworthy cases in the modern era. Jerry Wills is one such example. He made an impression on Rob Haberer, a broadcast-news producer who has "helped expose fakes and frauds preying on people in need."[10] Jerry's work was so impressive to him that he wrote a book about him titled *Healer: The Jerry Wills Story* (2012). Haberer writes: "I'm still a skeptic by training and by nature....All I know is that most of the people Jerry works on are suddenly better. Their pain is gone."[11] The story of one of Jerry's miracle healings was featured on FOX in 2006, and the clip is available today on YouTube.[12]

Or consider the case of Dr. and Master Sha who is certified in Chinese healing modalities and earned a medical degree in Western medicine. Dr. Sha caught the attention of Yale- and Harvard-trained author William Gladstone. In his book *Miracle Soul Healer* (2011), Gladstone chronicles his journey to understand Dr. Sha's work. He writes: "How could reports of instant healings of deafness, cancer, lupus, back injuries, and knee injuries be true? How could the reports of his ability to empower others to also perform healings be true? I was determined to discover the truth or falsehood of this mystery. I left no stone unturned....I interviewed dozens of Dr. Sha's students, scores of whom he had claimed to heal."[13] Gladstone's thorough research revealed astounding results. He writes in the concluding chapter of his book: **"Thousands and perhaps tens of thousands of soul healing miracles by Dr. Sha [and his trained healers] have already occurred....I am absolutely certain that Dr. Sha's soul healing miracles are real."**[14] [emphasis added]

How does Dr. Sha do it? The wisdom that has enabled his healing abilities has come in part from his encounters with "the Divine." This is a far cry from anything remotely allopathic. Through whatever mechanism Dr. Sha obtained this knowledge, it has no doubt contributed to tangible, positive results.

For instance, one message Dr. Sha received was about a "spiritual law" that is as follows: "Everyone, including everything, is a universal servant to share universal love, forgiveness, peace, healing, blessing, harmony, and enlightenment....If one offers a little service, receive a little reward from the universe and [the Divine]. If one offers unconditional service, receive unlimited rewards."[15]

Thus, Dr. Sha ultimately espouses "karma cleansing" as an essential mechanism for performing miracles.[16] This ethos led to the development of an exercise that enables powers of healing and transformation. As Gladstone summarizes it: "You forgive all those who may have harmed you in this or past lifetimes. You must not just forgive them totally, but you must honor and appreciate those who have harmed you."[17] The notion that healing energy could be derived from emotional shifts is a fundamental insight (more on this soon).

Furthermore, Dr. Sha makes revelatory statements about the nature of the human being: "Soul is a light being. A human being is made of jing qi shen [pronounced *jing chee shun*]. Jing is matter. Qi is energy. Shen is soul. They are three elements, but they are also one."[18]

The fact that Dr. Sha holds such a perspective while being able to perform miracle healings—and can teach others to do so—is yet another demonstration of how much modern allopathic medicine is missing with its reductionistic, physicalist outlook.

The Biofield

Miracle healings raise many questions about how the body fundamentally works. Dr. Shamini Jain explores this notion in her book *Healing Ourselves: Biofield Science and the Future of Health* (2021). She writes:

> We are bioelectromagnetic beings. We often don't think about our bodies in terms of electricity and magnetism. We have been schooled to think of our human bodies as bags of bones, organs, muscles, liquids, and chemicals. But the truth is that humans, as with all living beings, absorb and emit energy....
>
> Scientific studies have explored how the biofield of a person interacts with the biofield of the Earth and what the Earth-human connection can mean for our health....
>
> Researchers [have] found, via controlled experiments, that altering the geomagnetic field [of Earth] actually influenced human brainwaves. Not only do geomagnetic fluctuations affect our brains, but they also appear to influence our heart rhythms.
>
> Ancient understandings of subtle energy form the basis of many medical traditions worldwide that fit under the biofield umbrella. The term *biofield* helps us bridge ancient and contemporary understandings of our bioelectromagnetic bodies and provide a common language for practice and research that explore and focus on the body's energy fields for health. The biofield perspective takes us beyond an understanding of our bodies as machines—separated from each other—to seeing them as bioenergetic beings deeply intertwined with our environments.[19]

One might then wonder how increased electricity and electromagnetic radiation are impacting our health in unseen ways.

The implications extend into healing practices too. Dr. Jain led a study, published in *Cancer* in 2011, in which breast-cancer survivors who received a biofield healing experienced less fatigue and improved hormonal function compared to those in control groups.[20] She comments in her book:

> What floored me was the effectiveness of the treatment. These breast cancer survivors were selected because they

> had high levels of fatigue that wouldn't go away even after treatment—some of them had been suffering with that fatigue for up to ten years. Yet, when compared with members of the waitlist control group, who went on with their lives and treatments as usual, the levels of fatigue in the women in the healing group dropped to what you would expect for a regular person down the street—their fatigue remitted to completely normal levels in a month's time, after only eight one-hour healing sessions. This was not only a statistically significant effect but also a highly significant clinical effect.[21]

The healers insist, however, that they are not the true healers but rather are facilitating the realignment with one's soul or spirit and clearing stuck energy in the person's biofield.[22] Their method was to lay their hands on patients' feet and legs and try to "stimulate bone-marrow chi" (*chi* is a word for energy in Chinese medicine, similar to *prana* in Indian medicine, and to various "subtle" energies described in other traditions). They also focused on detecting balances and imbalances within the patient's biofield to create an energetic flow where it had been blocked. This process, according to the healers, helps to release toxicity.[23]

Dr. Jain also examined biofield healing studies in addition to her own and found positive results—the healing modality can reduce pain intensity, and it even affects biological markers.[24]

A related modality is that of tuning-fork healing. Eileen Day McKusick, a practitioner of this modality, sums up the way she believes it works in her book *Electric Body, Electric Health* (2021): "The human body is not only an instrument, it is a self-tuning instrument. Just like you can use a tuning fork to tune a piano or guitar, somewhat miraculously, you can also use a tuning fork to tune the body.... Through the introduction of the coherent sound input of the tuning fork, chaotic waveforms come to a more harmonious expression."[25]

There are other nontraditional modalities that also seem to promote healing, such as yoga, meditation, qigong, and tai chi.

They all potentially relate to the human biofield and the body's energetic structure. In her book, Dr. Jain aggregates study after study suggesting that these modalities really do something. The studies suggest that yoga reduces pain and depression as well as fatigue in cancer survivors; it reduces fatigue in patients with multiple sclerosis; and reduces headaches and menopausal symptoms.[26] Studies also show that mindfulness meditation programs reduce the experience of pain, help with mental health, can reduce emotional suffering in cancer patients, and even impact the brain.[27] Similarly, the bodily movements in qigong and tai chi have been shown to lower blood pressure, improve the functioning of those with chronic disease, help cancer patients with sleep and fatigue, and reduce inflammation.[28]

Modern science may not yet understand *how* all of this works, but the effects are important, nonetheless. These concepts must be incorporated into a comprehensive paradigm of medicine.

Invisible Interconnectedness and Resonance

Embedded within concepts like the biofield and energy healing is a deeper notion of interconnectivity. This is implied by the metaphysics of the One Mind, in which all individual minds are connected within a broader "stream." It's also compatible with the notion of quantum entanglement.[29]

There even seems to be an ability for humans to harmonize their physiological states, which can be seen in the work of the HeartMath Institute. The organization's 2015 book *Science of the Heart* summarizes its years of scientific research, led by Rollin McCraty, PhD. The book states: "We have found that synchronization of heart-rhythm patterns between individuals is possible.... We have found that individuals who have a close working or living relationship are the best candidates for exhibiting true heart-rhythm synchronization."[30] For instance, in one study, two women who have a close relationship were asked to consciously focus on appreciating one another while sitting four feet apart, and their heart rates synchronized.[31] Heart-rate synchronization can also occur during sleep among couples in a stable and loving long-term relationship.[32]

Also, as noted by Larry Dossey, MD, twins can experience identical or similar thoughts and have physical changes at the same time. Dr. Dossey elaborates, mentioning a case of four-year-old female twins:

> The father took one of his little girls off to visit the grandparents several kilometers away. The other little girl didn't want to go. She stayed home to help her mother with household chores. Well, in so doing, she touched a red-hot iron and immediately erupted in a big fat second-degree blister—second-degree burn—on her hand. And as it turns out, the other little twin girl....at the grandparents' house several kilometers away, erupted at the same moment in an identical burn, on the same hand—the same part of the hand—[with] the same pattern. This was investigated by a doctor and a research team for the University of Madrid....Not all identicals have this, and only about 20 or 30 percent of them describe this. The fact is that a lot of identical twins don't enjoy being identical.[33]

Dr. Dossey also addresses the bigger-picture significance: "The key in all of these cases seems to be emotional closeness....This spreads beyond twins. A lot of people can be emotionally close and aren't twins, such as lovers and parents, and just plain old friends. And so these are the people who describe these things. They are quite sensational. I don't know any way to ascribe these events to chance. To me that's just going too far. I think that there's something about emotional bonding that sets the stage for these events across great distances that just can hardly be explained in any other way."[34]

Emotional bonding might also relate to our connection to Earth's "field." As summarized by HeartMath's president and CEO, Deborah Rozman, PhD:

> Studies were done with groups of participants wearing heart-rate variability (HRV) recorders over long

> periods of time to determine how the solar and earth magnetic fields affect autonomic nervous system functioning. One surprising finding was that certain solar radio changes and lower magnetic field disturbances evoked a positive nervous system response. Mental clarity increased and people felt better.
>
> An even more surprising finding from the data was an indication that participants' heart rhythms were synchronizing at a deep level to some external signal in the earth's magnetic-field environment. What was found was that participants who were thousands of miles away from each other showed synchronized HRV. One hypothesis is that the magnetic field of the earth... is somehow connecting people in sync. The magnetic field is the medium. What the data implies is that we are both receiving information from the magnetic field and feeding information into the field. **The evidence suggests that what tunes us to the field is emotional bonding. That the primary determinant of how in sync we are with each other regardless of distance is our emotional bonding.**[35] [emphasis added]

Many speculative ideas come to mind here. The potential importance of electromagnetism on health is one of them. But also, the notion of emotional bonding and being "in sync" carries with it many implications. One might wonder if being "in sync" can influence manifestations of health and disease—almost like a nonphysical, non-germ-based "contagion." In other words, is there an energetic "resonance" between people whereby aspects of one person's state transfers to the other's "biofield"? Do we "broadcast" something when we are sick, whereby someone else would pick up the signal and perhaps align with it if they're not "protecting their energy field"? Can one person's detoxification process—manifesting as symptoms of "illness"—rub off on others energetically, thereby causing them to have similar symptoms?

The implications extend into other biological life as well. For instance, the work of former CIA lie-detection expert Cleve Backster is instructive with respect to what he called "biocommunication."[36] To his great surprise, he found in 1966 that when he hooked up his plant to one of his polygraph machines, the plant responded to his *intent* to burn one of its leaves.[37] As he wrote in his book *Primary Perception* (2003): "The very moment the imagery of burning that leaf entered my mind, the polygraph recording pen moved rapidly to the top of the chart! No words were spoken, no touching the plant, no lighting of matches, just my clear intention to burn the leaf. The plant recording showed dramatic excitation."[38]

As he continued his experimentation over several years, he concluded that "there had to be a real intent to do something harmful in order to observe the chart reaction. If you merely pretended, you would not cause a reaction. The plant seemed to know when you didn't mean it. They appeared to pick up the difference between your pretense and your true intent."[39]

His studies went beyond plants, however. He experimented on a "just matured" batch of kombucha—a fermented tea that contains live bacteria. Backster had begun researching kombucha and commented, "I became...intrigued when I read statements...that seemed to personalize the relationship between kombucha and its users—such as, it should be given away, never sold, and if you talk to it nicely, you will get a better beverage. Some users claim that it is also sensitive to negativity in the environment."[40] He then hooked up a new batch of kombucha to his machine, and he found that it responded to an intense emotional response he had while watching the movie *Conspiracy Theory*, starring Mel Gibson and Julia Roberts, which he hadn't previously seen. The living organisms in the kombucha had a "large reaction." The spike occurred during the part of the movie that reminded Backster of particularly sensitive aspects of his CIA experience (which related to the use of hallucinogens and sensory deprivation in CIA experiments).[41] The implication is that the living material in the kombucha responded to his heightened emotional state.

One might wonder: Can this happen between humans? And could the phenomenon end up creating something that people misinterpret as germ-based contagion, whereby one person's sickness causes a physiological change in someone else (via an unseen energetic connection)?

In another instance, Backster had hooked up electrodes to a container of yogurt (which had live bacteria). He took some of the yogurt from the electrode source and placed it in a separate beaker. Then he dropped into the beaker a form of powdered penicillin, which kills bacteria. He found that the source from which that yogurt came—the container that was hooked up to electrodes—showed "a huge reaction." The implication is that the yogurt in the original source could sense that "members of its family" (to speak in metaphor) were being killed by antibiotics.[42]

One might wonder: Does this happen to humans? If lots of people are getting sick, could it cascade because people energetically pick up the negative emotions?

Backster also experimented with human white blood cells. He took samples, hooked them up to electrodes, and observed whether the mental state of the person from whom he had taken the cells impacted the cells. For instance, while one man's cells were outside of his body, hooked up to electrodes, he was flipping through a *Playboy* magazine. While the man looked at the centerfold picture of a nude model, Backster reported that the man's "in vitro white cells showed [a] full-scale reaction, hitting the top and bottom limit stops on the chart recorder."[43] The cells were *outside* of his body. Backster continued, "After two full minutes of continuous reactivity, I suggested that he close the magazine. When [the man] closed the magazine, his electrode cells calmed down as he attempted a process of mental dissociation. Then, a minute later, when he reached over to again open the closed magazine, the cells spiked again. When [the man] experienced this high-quality observation, knowing his feelings and the thoughts in his own mind, it was the end of any raw skepticism about our research."[44]

Backster also noted that the CIA replicated his work on human cells in vitro: "The replication was successful, and it was during this period that high-quality observations were made of human cell biocommunication over a distance of twelve miles. Less-structured observations involved a distance in excess of fifty miles."[45]

Moreover, the work of psychoneuroimmunologist Dr. Paul Pearsall is potentially related to such phenomena. In his book *The Heart's Code* (1999), he described instances in which organ-transplant recipients became linked in consciousness to the donor. In one instance, an eight-year-old girl who had received a heart transplant began having nightmares about a murder. It was so severe that her parents took her to a psychiatrist. The young girl provided details of the murder and the murderer. As it turns out, the eight-year-old girl had received the heart of a ten-year-old girl who had been murdered, and somehow the memories were transmitted via the donated heart. According to Dr. Pearsall, the psychiatrist brought the details of the murder to the police, and they were able to find and arrest the murderer of the heart donor.[46]

In another instance, a fifty-two-year-old man who had received a transplanted heart from a seventeen-year-old boy began to love loud rock music after having previously enjoyed classical music. He was married, but began fantasizing about teenage girls. In other words, he began to take on characteristics of the heart donor.[47]

Also, a thirty-five-year-old woman who received the heart of a forty-two-year-old prostitute began experiencing significant changes in her sex drive. She began doing things that she says she "would never have done" before her surgery. Testimony provided by her husband validated this. He reported: "Not that I'm complaining, mind you, but what I have now is a sex kitten."[48]

But it's not just the heart that has these qualities. Dr. Pearsall described the case of a kidney recipient who began craving spicy foods such as tacos and burritos, even though, historically, he hadn't enjoyed spicy foods. He also started taking Spanish classes. It turned out that the kidney he received had come from a young Hispanic man.[49]

Modern allopathic medicine does not account for anything like the discussed phenomena. There appears to be a hidden interconnectedness and resonance—not only between living beings but also between the component parts of living beings—as well as between living beings and electromagnetic characteristics of Earth. These factors seem like essential considerations when trying to uncover the causes of disease and the determinants of health.

Spontaneous Healing and Consciousness Shifts

There are many documented cases of sudden healing that would be impossible, according to allopathic medicine. A relevant compendium, published in 1993, was developed by Marilyn Schlitz, PhD, at the Institute of Noetic Sciences. A summary of the remarkable analysis is as follows:

> Spontaneous remission [refers to] "the disappearance, complete or incomplete, of a disease or cancer without medical treatment or treatment that is considered inadequate to produce the resulting disappearance of disease symptoms or tumor." Because there was [previously] no standard reference for the field of spontaneous remission..., the first task of the Remission Project at [the Institute of Noetic Sciences] was to catalogue the world's medical literature on the subject. **As a result, it assembled the largest database of medically reported cases of spontaneous remission in the world, with more than 3,500 references from more than 800 journals in 20 different languages.**
>
> While the authors believe that the phenomenon of remission is relatively rare, the data from their research suggest that it may not be as rare as previously believed. It appears that the impression of rarity is at least partly an artifact of underreporting.[50] [emphasis added]

A more recent case—one that has received significant attention—is that of Anita Moorjani. After four years of suffering from cancer, she was in a terminal state and had to be rushed to the hospital in 2006. The doctor told her husband, "Your wife's heart may still be beating...but she's not really there. It's too late to save her. Her organs have already shut down. Her tumors have grown to the size of lemons throughout her lymphatic system, from the base of her skull to below her abdomen. Her brain is filled with fluid, as are her lungs. And as you can see, her skin has developed lesions that are weeping with toxins. She won't even make it through the night."[51]

She then had a profound NDE that ultimately changed the course of her life entirely. The details are startling, but typical of what near-death experiencers often report:

> Although I try to share my near-death experience... there are no words that can come close to describing its depth and the amount of knowledge that came flooding through....
>
> Imagine, if you will, a huge, dark warehouse. You live there with only one flashlight to see by. Everything you know about what's contained within this enormous space is what you've seen by the beam of one small flashlight. Whenever you want to look for something, you may or may not find it, but that doesn't mean the thing doesn't exist. It's there, but you just haven't shone your light on it....
>
> That is what physical life is like. We're only aware of what we focus our senses on at any given time, and we can only understand what is already familiar.
>
> Next, imagine that one day, someone flicks on a switch. There for the first time, in a sudden burst of brilliance and sound and color, you can see the entire warehouse, and it's nothing like anything you'd ever imagined. Lights are blinking, flashing, glowing, and shooting sparks of red, yellow, blue, and green. You see colors you don't recognize, ones you've never seen before. Music

> floods the room with fantastic, kaleidoscopic, surround-sound melodies you've never heard before. Neon signs pulse and boogie in rainbow strobes.[52]

Moorjani thus came to appreciate that "what you used to think was your reality was, in fact, hardly a speck within the vast wonder that surrounds you." She began to see "how all the various parts are interrelated, how they all play off each other, how everything fits."[53]

While in this "other realm," as she calls it, Moorjani met the spirit of her deceased father. She felt "unconditional love"[54] for him in spite of the pressure she felt from him while he was living. She then had a realization that changed her life: **"I understood that my body is only a reflection of my internal state.** If my inner self were aware of its greatness and connection with All-that-is, my body would soon reflect that and heal rapidly. To access this state of allowing, the only thing I had to do was be myself! I realized that all those years, all I ever had to do was be myself, without judgment or feeling that I was flawed." Her understanding was that "at the core, our essence is made of pure love. We are pure love—every single one of us....Therefore, being love and being our true self is one and the same thing!"[55] [emphasis added]

Moorjani then came out of her coma and proceeded to have a miracle recovery, which she attributes to this realization. It was a true shift in consciousness, and perhaps even an "energetic" upgrade. About six days after leaving the ICU, her doctors ran a test to examine the state of her cancer. One of them remarked: "I don't understand. I have scans that show this patient's lymphatic system was ridden with cancer just two weeks ago, but now I can't find a lymph node on her body large enough to even suggest cancer.... **Cancer doesn't just disappear like that**."[56] [emphasis added]

Moorjani has been healthy since this miracle healing, and she now speaks all over the world. And she's not the only one to have a miracle healing from an NDE—author David Sunfellow has aggregated numerous other cases.[57]

David Hawkins, MD, PhD, also experienced miracle healings (outside of an NDE context, however). In his book *Letting Go*

(2012), he listed two pages' worth of illnesses that he'd previously had. He said, "There were so many illnesses all at once that it was impossible to remember them all."[58] He had tried many alternative therapies, but it wasn't until he recognized that he needed to *shift his consciousness* that his conditions miraculously disappeared. **The ultimate solution was to allow himself to feel his emotions—fully—and let go of resisting them.**

He also let go of resisting the symptoms themselves. He wrote about the mindset shift he experienced when having "massive hemorrhaging" from diverticulitis:

> Instead of going to the hospital and getting transfusions, there was complete surrender. All of the sensations going on in the abdomen were acknowledged and not resisted. They were not given a name or a label. Instead of thoughts or words, there was a sense of oneness with the sensations, the cramps, and the pain. There was no resistance to the sensations, no matter how intense. Like being on a razor's edge, every sensation and feeling was recognized and surrendered. This went on for four solid hours. At the end of four hours, the bleeding stopped, the cramps went away, and the diverticulitis was healed. Later, there were some minor recurrences; but each one was handled in the same way, and eventually the attacks subsided and disappeared. So the mechanism of surrender passed the acid test. It succeeded where everything else had failed. With continued application, other disorders began to fade away.[59]

He wrote in summary: "It was discovered that there is a self-healing power *within* that is activated by continual surrender."[60]

Furthermore, he talked about the importance of one's beliefs in his book *Healing and Recovery* (2009). In his view:

> Mind is so powerful that it creates the thought form which manifests on the physical plane, thus becoming a physical reality. We can see that self-healing then really depends on the reversal of the usual belief

> systems of causality. What we hold in mind manifests on the physical level; it is not the other way around.... At the same time, we are letting go of the sources of unconscious guilt and stopping the reinforcement of the illnesses that come from labeling and propagating them, thereby bringing about a fulfillment of our own self-prophecies....We cannot allow the mind to come up with a belief system without challenging it.[61]

An emerging approach to healing, which also focuses on the mind, is known as German New Medicine (GNM). Its core principles were uncovered in the late 1970s by Dr. Ryke Geerd Hamer.[62] In particular, it focuses on "shock" events in one's life that manifest as ailments in the body—even cancer—which reflect the body's attempt to assist with the shock.

Thus, emotions are an essential element of health in GNM. Caroline Markolin, PhD, elaborates on this topic on her GNM-education website, https://learninggnm.com/:

> In GNM, the psyche is regarded as an integral part of the human biology. It is the "organ," so to speak, that inherently recognizes dangers. At the very instance of [an emotionally distressing event], the psyche associates with the event a specific biological conflict theme such as "anger in the territory," "worries in the nest," "abandonment by the pack," "separation from a mate," "loss of an offspring," and so forth. This association happens in a split second and entirely on a subliminal level. Thus, it is the subconscious reading and subjective assessment of the conflict situation that determines which Biological Special Program will be activated. Yet, how exactly the subconscious mind perceived the particular conflict is only revealed when the physical symptoms arise. **Whether a person gets a sore throat, comes down with a cold, has diarrhea, [or] develops a skin condition or a certain cancer is therefore dependent on how the conflict was experienced when the [emotionally distressing event] occurred....We can also**

> **suffer a conflict with or on behalf of someone else.**[63] [emphasis added]

Dr. Markolin notes that "with the resolution of the conflict, the autonomic nervous system switches," and steps toward healing can begin. But in GNM, a "track" can reactivate the emotional shock. A track could be "the location where the conflict took place, a person or pet that was involved, the taste of a particular food, specific sounds or noises, the weather condition, a certain scent (perfume, flowers), certain words, a voice, a gesture, and so forth." Dr. Markolin continues: "If we are in the healing phase and suddenly encounter a track, either through direct contact or by association, **the original conflict is instantly reactivated. Each conflict relapse interrupts and therefore prolongs the healing process—on the correlating organ as well as in the corresponding brain relay—leading to a chronic condition."**[64] [emphasis added]

Therefore, GNM highlights the *psychological* components of *physical* disease. The general idea is that traumas manifest as physical symptoms that traditional doctors label as specific conditions. But under GNM, symptoms reflect the body's process of healing. Moreover, from this lens, healing becomes viewed as an *internal* process that is the responsibility of the individual. This stands in stark contrast to the allopathic model, in which the individual's health is often dependent on pharmaceutical drugs to suppress symptoms.

The implications of this approach are further summarized by holistic psychiatrist Kelly Brogan, MD, in her 2023 interview with GNM practitioner Dr. Melissa Sell: "The paradigm shift that is required [is] to move from this idea that the symptoms of a so-called illness are the problem to resolve, to a paradigm that says the symptoms are evidence of resolution....When you say, 'actually, what we are experiencing as symptoms is the resolution—it's already underway,' now we can support your body in whatever way is necessary, and you can integrate that."[65]

From an even broader perspective, "disease" could be viewed as an evolutionary stimulus. It forces us to look within, and in so doing, we grow. Excessively suppressing symptoms, from this lens, could be counterproductive because it's a mere Band-Aid that stunts one's progress—possibly even on a "soul" level.

Beyond This Body and This Life

There's an even deeper level to "looking into the past" than what GNM describes. It involves considering potential "previous lives." In his exploration of children with past-life memories, the University of Virginia's Ian Stevenson, MD, found cases of children who had birthmarks or physical defects that aligned with the injury resulting in the death of the person in the previous life. Allopathic medicine typically views genetics and environment as the factors to consider in biological health and disease. **And yet the work that has emerged from the University of Virgina suggests that there is a "third factor" that needs to be accounted for.**[66]

In his book *Where Reincarnation and Biology Intersect* (1997), Dr. Stevenson wrote: "The birthmarks and birth defects provide an objective type of evidence well above that which depends on the fallible memories of informants. We have photographs (and occasionally sketches) which show the birthmarks and birth defects. And for many of the cases, we have a medical document, usually a postmortem report, that gives us written confirmation of the correspondence between the birthmark (or birth defect) and the wound on the deceased person whose life the child, when it can speak, will usually claim to remember."[67]

Dr. Stevenson also found that the children have specific phobias and philias (desires) that relate to the person from the previous life. He noted that phobias occur in about 35 percent of the cases. For instance, he wrote: "A child remembering a life that ended in drowning may be afraid of being immersed in water....If the death occurred during a vehicular accident, the subject may have a phobia of automobiles, buses, and trucks. These phobias often manifest before the child has begun to speak."[68] Dr. Stevenson mentioned that philias "frequently take the form of a desire or demand for particular foods (not eaten in the subject's family) or for clothes different from those customarily worn by family members. Under this heading also comes cravings for addicting substances, such as tobacco, alcohol, and other drugs that the previous personality was known to have used. A few subjects show skills they have not been taught (or sufficiently watched others demonstrating), but which the previous personality was known to have had."[69]

But past-life memories aren't limited to children. Some adults spontaneously remember them, but they can also be induced via hypnotic regression. It's not always a reliable method.

Sometimes, however, the results are astounding. In particular, consider the case of Mira Kelley. In an interview on Laura Powers's *Healing Powers* podcast in 2016, Kelley explained her personal story: She was an attorney who developed severe jaw pain (TMJ). The pain was so serious that she was unable to eat or sleep, and she was not finding solutions through traditional healing methods. Her doctor wanted to perform an operation that would break her jaw, which she didn't want to do. Alternatively, the doctor said she would have to live with chronic pain. So out of desperation, she worked with a past-life-regression specialist in the hopes of finding a nontraditional solution.

A memory emerged of a man's life in which he was a slave with a big chain around his neck. She felt his powerlessness, and it was "emotionally moving" to her. **The next morning her jaw pain was gone.** Eventually she stopped practicing law and became a past-life-regression therapist herself so that she could help others.[70]

There are also many instances of "between lives" memories. Sometimes they are accessed via hypnotic regression, but some children also remember them. More specifically, a subset of children who have previous-life memories also have memories of an "intermission" period before they entered their next bodies. These cases are summarized in a 2004 paper by the University of Virginia's Poonam Sharma and Jim Tucker, MD, published in the *Journal of Near-Death Studies*. The authors comment that intermission memories "can be broken down into three parts: a transitional stage [after death], a stable stage in a particular location, and a return stage involving choosing parents or conception."[71]

The notion of "choosing" elements of a life before birth is noteworthy in the context of medicine. In Robert Schwartz's book *Your Soul's Plan: Discovering the Real Meaning of the Life You Planned Before You Were Born* (2007), he's found that souls sometimes plan immense challenges—even physical ailments—before birth. Although on one level this seems masochistic, Schwartz's research has offered a more positive spin. He finds that prebirth agreements or contracts can be made whereby the planned challenges lead to growth on a soul level and ultimately induce a movement toward self-love.[72]

Along these lines, Serena Faith-Masterson's account is worth considering. She was born into a satanic cult, sold into a covert government mind-control program by her father, and developed more than 300 unique personalities because of the torture she endured.[73] But later in life she was able to heal, miraculously, and reintegrate the fragmented parts of her mind (with the help of a devoted healer). She writes in her book *I Am Serena* (2020): "My Soul...began to share with me the intent of this lifetime. Before my birth, my Soul knew of thousands of years she had lived in human form experiencing life through a veil of self-hatred. She chose that this lifetime would be different. By being born to parents who were masters of fear, I would create such an exaggerated experience of fear that I would either get lost in it, or I would discover the truth of who I really am. It was a big gamble, but my Soul was willing to take it."[74]

How should these various concepts be integrated into a more comprehensive view of healing? Might past lives and prebirth contracts play a role in our health in this life? If prebirth agreements occur, are they always made willingly, or, sometimes, can a soul be forced, coerced, or even deceived by "tricksters"? An incredibly complex picture emerges with the accumulation of such data points.

These alleged "past life" and "between lives" memories raise big questions not only about healing but also about memory. What's implied is that we humans live with amnesia with respect to other aspects of our deeper identity. Furthermore, memory isn't stored in the brain but rather is *accessed by* the brain (and perhaps other parts of the body, as seen in the cases of organ transplants). That's certainly not something contemplated in allopathic medicine.

Rupert Sheldrake, PhD, a former Cambridge biochemist, has explored this notion as it relates to a slightly different topic: collective memory. His theory of "morphic resonance" posits: "Memory need not be stored in material traces inside brains, which are more like TV receivers than video recorders, tuning into influences from the past. And biological inheritance need not all be coded in the genes, or in epigenetic modifications of the genes; much of it depends on morphic resonance from previous members of the species. **Thus each individual inherits a collective memory from past members of the species, and also contributes to the collective memory, affecting other members of the species in the future."**[75] [emphasis added]

This concept raises questions about the relationship between an individual and one's broader species—and the related implications for health and disease on a collective level. **If the mind can impact matter, and if there's a collective consciousness that we're tapping into, what happens when many people are in fear or are sick? Could it cascade because of the interconnectivity of the morphic field?**

Similarly, one might wonder if ancestral lines carry an energetic connection to an individual in ways not well understood by traditional medicine (though it is explored in "family constellation" therapy[76]).

Otherworldly Influences

Beyond "past life," "between lives," species-wide, or even ancestral influences on health, there's another consideration not covered within allopathic medicine: the notion that unseen forces are affecting us.

From a physicalist perspective, this doesn't make sense; but from the One Mind perspective, there could be multidimensional "whirlpools" in the same stream of consciousness that impact our own consciousness.

Some people are able to actively tap into these other energies via a process known as channeling. Helané Wahbeh's book *The Science of Channeling* (2021) describes the process by which nonphysical, intelligent entities can be "channeled" by a human, and the being speaks through the vocal cords of the human. That is, humans can willingly "call in" such beings. Many channelers, while channeling, speak differently than they normally do, and sometimes their body moves in strange ways. Wahbeh's research suggests that these instances are often distinct from what would be seen in individuals with a mental disorder. In fact, when people claim to be channeling, random-number generators placed in the same room behave nonrandomly.[77] This suggests that the channeler is indeed doing something authentic—at least sometimes.

Therefore, it's not a stretch to believe that we are all "channeling"—to some degree—constantly. That is, we're picking up energy, creativity, and even thoughts from forces beyond what we can see with our eyes. And the "antenna" of our brain/body system picks up the signal. How might such influences be affecting our mindset and our health?

Along these lines, demonic possession deserves consideration. In addition to religious traditions that report this phenomenon, Richard Gallagher, MD—a Princeton and Yale graduate and a professor of clinical psychiatry at New York Medical College—has personally experienced this with patients. He describes his path in his book *Demonic Foes: My Twenty-Five Years as a Psychiatrist Investigating Possessions, Diabolic Attacks, and the Paranormal* (2020).

The cases of possession he's examined were either sent to him by clergy, or they found him when they learned that he specializes in possession cases.[78] He decided to write the book because, in his words, "I want to enlighten the public as to the import and reality of these admittedly rare phenomena and what must be done for someone to receive help. I want to see tormented people set free from all things that would oppress or destroy their lives. I've dedicated my life to fighting the ravages of mental illness, and I've put the same sort of passion into working with people who may suffer from demonic possessions or lesser attacks, however controversial such conclusions may seem to some of my peers."[79]

He notes that possessions differ from "various psychoses and severe personality and dissociative disorders…in significant ways."[80] Dr. Gallagher mentions one case in particular that featured symptoms typical of possession, including "involuntary trance states; vitriolic expressions of hatred toward religion, delivered in a diabolic-sounding voice; and other paranormal abilities including speaking in Latin, a language that [the patient] did not know." He mentions that during exorcisms, the room can become frigid.[81]

Dr. Gallagher's conclusion is that "a segment of [the] invisible world seems to be mysteriously but remarkably hostile to human beings and seeks their physical and spiritual destruction. On rare occasions, like some kind of cosmic terrorist, that segment shows its true colors."[82] [emphasis added]

Father Chad Ripperger, a Catholic priest who performs exorcisms, provides additional insights based on his experience in dealing with demonic beings. His words imply a hierarchy of consciousness among nonphysical entities. For instance, in a 2023 lecture, he says that demons don't have a choice in terms of whom they possess:

> What that basically means is this. There are two types of possessions: there are possessions in which God permits them in the sense of, [God] says "You can possess this individual." And because demons [are] fixed on the evil, it's almost like they're compulsive. They'll just do it…. [But] there [are] other times where [God] says, "You *must* possess this person." Now that sounds strange. But then we call that conscription. And basically what it is, is God is allowing the possession. **And [God] tells them they have to possess the person because there's something in the person's life or through the possession that [God]…wants the family or the individual**

> **to come to knowledge of.** So for example, there...were two cases of sisters who were blood related. And they were possessed by some of the same possessors....And the reason it became clear that God basically conscripted them into possession was because of the fact that he wanted a particular generational spirit to be expunged from the family line. A lot of times the demons don't have any control over the matter....
>
> **One of the cases I'm working on now, one of the... low-level demons...he had never possessed anybody, and the reason God told him you have to possess this woman is because in her battle to get this thing out, she was going to reach [an extreme] level of holiness....So God uses [the demons] as instruments. [The demons] will admit as much....So they don't get to choose anything....God lets demons do what they do...for our sanctification ultimately."**[83] [emphasis added]

A broader point implied by Fr. Ripperger's work—which may apply outside of the extreme cases of demonic position—is that evil serves a purpose in our world. In one regard, it's horrific and causes suffering. But the paradox is that it stimulates growth. Just like working out at the gym can be painful, it also leads to muscle growth, strength, and resilience. The nuances embedded in the concept of "growth" might be beyond human comprehension, yet there is a human tendency to want to simplify things into black-and-white notions of "good" and "bad." Ultimately, the fact that nonphysical forces are involved is an essential piece of the puzzle.

In fact, ancient civilizations also talked about nonphysical forces, even in the context of disease. As described in *A History of Experimental Virology* (1991) by Alfred Grafe: "Ancient Greece and its religious concepts of nature...date back to the Egyptian and Babylonian cultures, i.e., approximately 4000 BC: Through the intervention of demons and gods, mankind was beset by maladies and pestilence."[84]

Furthermore, in my book *An End to Upside Down Contact* (2022), I describe a wide variety of evidence suggesting that we are not alone and that a spectrum of beings seem to coexist with us—some are benevolent, others are malevolent, and others are in between. The beings might be physical and/or multidimensional, even if we don't ordinarily see them with our eyes. In fact, contact with such beings seems to have occurred throughout human history, as expressed in ancient lore from cultures all over the world.

Recall that Dr. Sha encountered an apparently *benevolent* entity—"the Divine"—and it taught him lessons about the universe that he's been able to use to heal people. Similarly, Serena Faith-Masterson's healer, Norma Delaney, helped her reintegrate her more than 300 unique personalities in part by employing a breathing method. Delaney had learned the method of "compassionate" breath—in which one breathes the soul deep into the lower belly—years prior, when a being named Kwan Yin suddenly appeared to her and taught her the method.[85] In this instance, like Dr. Sha's, the information obtained from the being was objectively helpful and health-inducing.

Pulitzer Prize winner John Mack, MD (1929–2004), the former head of psychiatry at Harvard, also studied human contact with nonhuman intelligences. He came to the conclusion that we are not alone after studying many cases of people claiming to have been "abducted" and who'd had direct contact with beings. Generally, Mack didn't feel that they were making up their accounts. There are even reports in which people are miraculously healed of serious illnesses directly *by* alleged beings themselves, and they often use light as a healing tool.[86] Preston Dennett's 2019 book, *The Healing Power of UFOs: 300 True Accounts of People Healed by Extraterrestrials*, explores some of these allegations. (Note: The terms used to describe "other intelligences" can vary, whether they're called ETs, interdimensionals, time travelers, angels, aliens, beings of light, and so on. People might use different words to describe similar phenomena, even though those words can have a different meaning depending on who uses them.)

Additionally, researchers such as Paul Wallis (a former archdeacon of the Australian Anglican church) make observations about ancient scriptures from around the world. The texts—if they're read as history rather than mythology—seem to suggest that advanced intelligences *created* humans. That doesn't make them "God," per se; it simply implies that they had advanced capabilities within the broader One Mind context, of which we're all a part. If there is even a hint of truth to this concept, our view of human biology needs to be revised. More fundamentally, this raises an important point: an accurate history of our species, and our civilization, is needed before we can truly understand who and what we are.[87]

These various factors must be considered and explored further within a new medical paradigm. And abandoning the primitive and outdated physicalist metaphysics is an essential prerequisite.

CONCLUSION

WHAT'S AT STAKE

The reductionistic, allopathic model of medicine is deeply flawed and based on outdated assumptions. And it has turned modern health care into an establishment that all too often endangers the very patients it's supposed to help.

Medicine *should be* devoted to caring for people. It *should be* about a human-to-human connection in the process of healing. While some noble practitioners embody these ideals, the *overall system* has become a "medical-industrial complex": an intricate web of financial interests involving pharmaceutical companies, doctors, nurses, medical device/equipment suppliers, diagnostics companies, hospitals, medical schools, insurance companies, media companies, politicians, technology companies, scientific journals, and others.[1]

Those who pull the strings of this web have managed to control society's belief systems about health and disease; and about germs, infections, contagion, and vaccines. Modern medicine's core beliefs are often blindly accepted—and even defended—when there is great reason to challenge them. And yet they persist.

The medical-industrial complex not only steers society's belief systems but also the practice of medicine itself. Making money often takes precedence over healing, while a deeper spiritual orientation is lacking.

From a financial perspective, healing a person means losing a customer. Having people stay on long-term pharmaceutical medications is a much better outcome than identifying and solving the underlying problem that's causing symptoms. Thus, for the pharmaceutical industry, it makes sense to fund research on drugs and vaccines rather than uncovering how to empower people to stay healthy *on their own*. Certainly, the medical system has saved people from life-threatening conditions, but at the same time, it hasn't focused as much on how it could have prevented those people from becoming deathly ill in the first place. Overall, a chronically sick society is a better economic outcome for the medical-industrial complex than a healthy society is. **This dangerous mentality can persist *if* participants within "the system" act from a physicalist perspective that has lost sight of the greater "cosmic system" that connects us all. As such, a consciousness shift is essential.**

In the absence of this shift, hospitals have become factory-like; and doctors and nurses, often unknowingly, have transformed into cogs in a wheel. Perhaps they enter the system with good intentions and genuinely want to help people. But indoctrination takes hold quickly, and the prospect of going against the grain is harrowing and outright intimidating. Speaking out carries great risk, so it's easier to just play it safe, not make a fuss, and unquestioningly follow the protocols. Patients who have experienced this dynamic can attest without hesitation: **compassion in the mainstream medical system is sometimes conspicuously absent.** In part, this might be due to a flawed philosophical outlook, but it's also a symptom of an unhealthy society. Given how many sick people are flooding the system, it's often a practical challenge for health-care providers to treat each patient with appropriate care and attention.

With these dynamics at play, many health-care providers do not focus on providing holistic solutions. Stale and simplistic narratives about why people get sick have transformed into invincible dogmas such that the only solution to illness is a magical pharmaceutical bullet. In other words, an external source must be the savior, and the patient is a mere victim.

Uncovering the true determinants of health and disease has become secondary, whereas it should be the primary objective in a system truly focused on well-being. That's where health-care providers, in theory, should be directing their attention. In essence, allopathy often focuses on what's under the microscope, rather than what's within the "macroscope."[2]

New Zealand surgeon-turned-naturopath Ulrich Williams saw this clearly back in 1937. He suggested basic principles that can redirect our current paradigm—and the thinking that underlies it—into something much better:

> The orthodox healing system has failed for reasons that easily can be defined....We have failed because from our too narrow and materialistic outlook we have conceived of disease as something attacking us from without, due to germs; whereas disease whether of body, mind, soul, or estate, is mostly a gradual degenerative process going on within, due to failure to comply with the requirements of well-being. We fail because in the zones of physical limit we look outside ourselves for cause and cure of troubles arising within. We have failed because the whole complicated system of orthodox modern diagnosis and treatment is based upon a misconception that mistakes the symptom for the disease; and tinkering with effects while the cause is ignored and allowed to continue always has been and will be followed by deplorable consequences.[3]

Furthermore, moving toward a better system of medicine might require looking back at ancient methods from a variety of cultures all over the world. Dr. Shamini Jain mentions Indian Ayurvedic, classical Chinese, and Tibetan teachings in particular, summarizing their approach and the implications thereof:

> The body has an innate ability to heal itself, and this process can be encouraged by fostering proper flow of

> life force energy, which serves as a conduit between consciousness and physicality.
>
> These Eastern teachings provide an underlying model to help us better understand and explore communications between the spirit, the body, and our environment. Disease is considered disharmony that might exist within one's self or between one's self and his or her surrounding environment. Thus, healing is not about curing yourself from something that is "not you" but understanding the patterns that might be causing you disharmony and therefore illness. The vital life force is a bridge that allows the healer—ultimately you—to better understand the nature of that disharmony and bring harmony back to your system.[4]

While we may not yet know *exactly* what a new paradigm of medicine will look like, at least we know what it *won't* look like.[5] Armed with a general compass for rethinking heath care, we have an opportunity to create a brighter future—both on an individual and collective level.

From the perspective of an individual, if we want to be healthy, it's simply not wise to rely exclusively on the mainstream allopathic system and its health-care providers (perhaps outside of emergency situations). Finding real health solutions requires reconsidering the basic nature of disease.

In their book *What Really Makes You Ill?*, Dawn Lester and David Parker lay out what they consider to be the four determinants of illness:[6]

1. Nutrition
2. Toxic exposures
3. Electromagnetic radiation
4. Stress

Notice that they don't focus on germs. Thus, from this perspective, "symptoms" reflect the body's attempt to heal or detoxify from an underlying ailment in one of those categories. Modern labels of discrete diseases are in many ways arbitrary distinctions for varying symptoms. Those labels often tell us nothing about the real *causes* of those symptoms.

An even broader way to think about it, in my view, is that ill health comes from:

1. Physical injury and/or
2. Psychospiritual injury

The first category can be a physical ailment (from, say, sports), but it also can relate to other aspects of physicality such as poor diet, environmental toxicity, electromagnetic toxicity, and so on. The second category relates to one's mental state, unresolved trauma, belief systems, emotions, "spiritual" connection, a sense of purpose in life, and even multidimensional matters that we don't fully understand.

What, then, should we do to stay healthy? Holistic practitioners might vary in their specific recommendations—such as detoxification protocols, dietary recommendations, herb and/or supplement recommendations, electromagnetic-protection solutions, body-alignment and somatic modalities, spiritual-practice suggestions, and so forth. But there seem to be some basic lifestyle recommendations, that they suggest across the board, which anyone can implement, such as eating nutritious and clean food; drinking clean water; avoiding toxins; sleeping well; exercising; getting sunlight and fresh air; avoiding excessive electromagnetic radiation; minimizing toxic forms of light (such as blue light from electronic screens); spending time in nature; having positive relationships; working on processing and clearing trauma; practicing forgiveness; feeling emotions rather than suppressing them; setting appropriate boundaries in relationships; laughing; following passions and joy; experiencing gratitude; being authentic; engaging in centering practices like meditation or breathing exercises; feeling a strong spiritual connection; discovering and following one's "soul purpose"; giving, receiving, and embodying love; and so on.[7] Maintaining good health might be much simpler than we've been led to believe by a pharmaceutical-dominated paradigm. These basic practices, which are empowering and largely inexpensive, enable independence from the overarching societal power structure. **Personal sovereignty isn't possible without taking the reins over one's own health.**

On a collective level, this is an essential point. We saw during the COVID-19 era that a "crisis" can be used as a pretext for taking citizens' rights away. What better way to control the global population than to bring about massive amounts of health-related fear—even for imaginary causes—wherein the only solution is the remedy provided by the authorities. The weaponization of fear around climate change has been taking on a similar quality.[8]

In fact, both are central pieces of the World Economic Forum's "Great Reset"—which was formally announced in June 2020 by Klaus Schwab and then–Prince Charles, and was described, in detail, in Schwab and Thierry Malleret's July 2020 book *COVID-19: The Great Reset*. As discussed in my book *An End to the Upside Down Reset* (2023), COVID-19 presented an opportunity to reset all aspects of society in a manner that a small number of people consider to be ideal. Perhaps the most significant point about the Great Reset is that it's not an agenda that emphasizes liberty or human flourishing; rather, it's much more focused on limiting freedom under the guise of "compassion." **Thus, we are currently living through an attempted reshaping of society, and *medicine* is one of the key levers that's being used to usher it in.**

As I've often contended, these matters extend beyond physical concerns; they are part of what appears to be a "spiritual war." One might wonder if the corrupt dynamics of the medical-industrial complex trace their roots to nonphysical forces of evil—the ultimate "string-pullers," invisible to our ordinary perceptual abilities. Such forces are drawn to power, and they seem to thrive off of the suffering of others; perhaps they even feed off of negative energy. Thus, the notions of eugenics and depopulation—in other words, culling the population like cattle—doesn't seem like a stretch. A medical system that's ostensibly supposed to save people, but in fact ends up harming them, is the perfect instrument for such an objective. And furthermore, a weakened and unhealthy populace is much easier to control than a strong and healthy one.

Even transhumanism—merging humans with artificial intelligence and altering our natural form—is often being promoted. The spiritual impact of such activities on the bodily vessel might be more hazardous than scientists currently acknowledge.

On a related note, in 1917 the mystic Rudolf Steiner foresaw the following:

> The time will come—and it may not be far off—when...people will say: It is pathological for people to even think in terms of spirit and soul. "Sound" people will speak of nothing but the body. It will be considered a sign of illness for anyone to arrive at the idea of any such thing as a spirit or a soul.... **The soul will be made nonexistent with the aid of a drug. Taking a "sound point of view," people will invent a vaccine to influence the organism as early as possible, preferably as soon as it is born, so that this human body never even gets the idea that there is a soul and a spirit....**
>
> **I have told you that the spirits of darkness are going to inspire their human hosts, in whom they will be dwelling, to find a vaccine that will drive all inclination towards spirituality out of people's souls when they are very young.**[9] [emphasis added]

The dystopian books *Brave New World* and *1984* no longer seem like fictional possibilities for our future—and from a metaphysical perspective, such enslavement could have even greater consequences than we know.

Dr. Anthony Fauci has openly discussed a "next pandemic."[10] Future global health scares seem inevitable, and COVID-19 showed us that the world can be shut down in an instant if the authority figures choose to do so. People's livelihoods can be determined on the basis of whether they take an experimental injection or not. A "positive" result on an unreliable test can lead to a mandatory quarantine sentence. Quarantine camps were even built as a result of COVID-19.[11]

Therefore, with such high stakes, discernment is essential; our ability to identify "wolves in sheep's clothing" needs to be sharp. A big piece of that is seeing through the dangers and falsities of the allopathic system, upon which many control mechanisms in society are based. That entails breaking out of the hypnotic spell of conditioned belief systems and engaging in independent, critical thinking rather than parroting the opinions of "experts." From a higher perspective, this process could be viewed as "evolutionary": in order for us to transcend the darkness of our world, we must be able to accurately perceive deception and navigate accordingly. We must learn to see through "false light." Therefore, the evil forces within the spiritual war either stimulate our growth and make us stronger (if we are able to catch on); or, if we don't, they'll consume us.

During his near-death experiences decades ago, Dannion Brinkley, the author of *Saved by the Light* (1994), was shown hints about our society's future. As he summarizes the message in a 2023 interview: **"I've been saying this for forty-eight years: the battle of humanity will be fought in health care."**[12] [emphasis added]

The question then arises: How should we approach this battle? Thomas Friese provides sound guidance in his 2013 preface to Ernst Jünger's *The Forest Passage* (1951). May these words echo in our consciousness as we navigate the treacherous waters ahead:

> The forces seeking to exploit man today are but the latest incarnations of forces that have threatened individual freedom throughout history....
>
> While [an individual's journey to freedom] may bring collateral benefits for society, in particular for other individuals, it does not aim primarily at world-improvement: the collective, as a whole, is essentially beyond redemption, a priori a lost cause. It is only individuals,...rebels

within society, that can hope, as exceptions, to escape the coercion, to "save their own souls." The...rebel[s] [battle] the Leviathan not in the hopes of defeating it—for it eventually collapses under its own enormous weight—though [they] may promote this inevitable demise by inflicting strategic damage on it, and [they] can already help define and introduce the seeds of new freedoms for a post-Leviathan world. Rather, the... rebel[s] [have] two other immediate motivations in the here and now: first, to save [themselves]...and second, and not unrelated, to obey [their] conscience...which feels natural concern for its fellow human beings.[13]

ACKNOWLEDGMENTS

Thank you to my publishers, Bill and Gayle Gladstone, of Waterside Productions, who have been so supportive of my writing journey. I also thank those who have assisted me in the process of publishing this book: Jill Kramer (copyediting/proofreading), Joel Chamberlain (design), Ken Fraser (cover art), Jennifer Uram (contract support), Sandi Schroeder (index), and Justin Levy (audiobook).

Thanks also to Dr. Andrew Kaufman and Dr. Mark Bailey for taking the time to review my manuscript and provide helpful feedback, and to Alec Zeck for his support throughout this process. More generally, I thank the many brave doctors and scientists who have been instrumental in questioning the prevailing narrative in order to usher in a new and improved paradigm. Thanks, as well, to the many healers who have helped me over the years. Finally, I am always appreciative of my friends and family for their continued encouragement and feedback.

ENDNOTES

OPENING QUOTATION

1 Sowell, *Economic Facts and Fallacies*, vii.

INTRODUCTION: ALLOPATHIC MEDICINE AND THE HURDLES TO OVERCOMING IT

1 CDC, "Chronic Diseases in America," https://www.cdc.gov/chronicdisease/resources/infographic/chronic-diseases.htm.
2 Ahmad et al., "Provisional Mortality Data — United States, 2022" https://www.cdc.gov/mmwr/volumes/72/wr/mm7218a3.htm.
3 Dalen et al., "The epidemic of the 20(th) century: coronary heart disease," https://pubmed.ncbi.nlm.nih.gov/24811552/.
4 National Cancer Institute, "National Cancer Act of 1971," https://dtp.cancer.gov/timeline/flash/milestones/M4_Nixon.htm.
5 Shenton, *Positively False*, 32.
6 Ahmad et al., "Provisional Mortality Data — United States, 2022" https://www.cdc.gov/mmwr/volumes/72/wr/mm7218a3.htm.
7 For instance, see the following publication by Johns Hopkins University: "Johns Hopkins study suggests medical errors are third-leading cause of death in U.S.," https://hub.jhu.edu/2016/05/03/medical-errors-third-leading-cause-of-death/. Also see Gussak et al., *Iatrogenicity: Causes and Consequences of Iatrogenesis in Cardiovascular Medicine*, chapter 5, https://www.jstor.org/stable/j.ctt1q1cr8b; and Makary and Daniel, "Medical error-the third leading cause of death in the US," https://pubmed.ncbi.nlm.nih.gov/27143499/.

8 Peer and Shabir, "Iatrogenesis: A review on nature, extent, and distribution of healthcare hazards," https://www.ncbi.nlm.nih.gov/pmc/articles/PMC6060929/.
9 Null, *Death by Medicine*, 36.
10 Engelbrecht et al., *Virus Mania*, 66.
11 Lipton, "THINK Beyond Your Genes – September 2021," https://www.brucelipton.com/think-beyond-your-genes-september-2021/. The discussion in the text about genetic determinism is not intended to suggest that no doctors think outside of the deterministic framework. Certainly, there are some who do, and the number of such practitioners is likely increasing. However, I'm pointing out a more general trend and attitude that views patients as mere victims of their circumstances rather than empowered individuals who can overcome hurdles. This is part of a reductionistic mindset that seems to bias the mentality within the mainstream, allopathic medical model.
12 AetherMedia22 Tony Punch, "Dr. Suzanne Humphries Lecture on Vaccines & Health! MY ADVICE YOU DIDNT ASK FOR, PAY CLOSE ATTENTION TO THIS ONE!!!," https://rumble.com/v24n1vi-dr.-suzanne-humphries-lecture-on-vaccine-and-health-my-advice-pay-close-att.html.
13 Sanexa, "New study shared by NIH suggests N95 Covid masks create dangerous of level toxic compounds linked seizures, cancer," https://www.bizpacreview.com/2023/08/27/new-study-shared-by-nih-suggests-n95-covid-masks-create-dangerous-of-level-toxic-compounds-linked-seizures-cancer-1390631/.
14 The Ring of Fire, "Big Pharma Owns Corporate Media, and It's Killing People," https://www.youtube.com/watch?v=q3lviBkaEUc.
15 Johns Hopkins Bloomberg School of Public Health, "Spending on Consumer Advertising for Top-Selling Prescription Drugs in U.S. Favors Those With Low Added Benefit," https://publichealth.jhu.edu/2023/spending-on-consumer-advertising-for-top-selling-prescription-drugs-in-us-favors-those-with-low-added-benefit.
16 The document mentions only the Carnegie Foundation in the copyright and the introduction. However, the association with Rockefeller Foundation is well known. For example, see "The Flexner Report—100 Years Later" by Thomas Duffy, MD, https://www.ncbi.nlm.nih.gov/pmc/articles/PMC3178858/.
17 Flexner, *Medical Education in the United States and Canada*, 158.
18 Duffy, "The Flexner Report—100 Years Later," https://www.ncbi.nlm.nih.gov/pmc/articles/PMC3178858/.
19 Hensley, "Big pharma pours millions into medical schools — here's how it can impact education," https://globalnews.ca/news/5738386/canadian-medical-school-funding/.
20 Ibid.
21 Ibid.

22 AetherMedia22 Tony Punch, "Dr. Suzanne Humphries Lecture on Vaccines & Health! MY ADVICE YOU DIDNT ASK FOR, PAY CLOSE ATTENTION TO THIS ONE!!!," https://rumble.com/v24n1vi-dr.-suzanne-humphries-lecture-on-vaccine-and-health-my-advice-pay-close-att.html.
23 White, "Why is the FDA Funded in Part by the Companies It Regulates?" https://today.uconn.edu/2021/05/why-is-the-fda-funded-in-part-by-the-companies-it-regulates-2/#.
24 Foley, "Trust issues deepen as yet another FDA commissioner joins the pharmaceutical industry," https://qz.com/1656529/yet-another-fda-commissioner-joins-the-pharmaceutical-industry.
25 Facher, "More than two-thirds of Congress cashed a pharma campaign check in 2020, new STAT analysis shows," https://www.statnews.com/feature/prescription-politics/federal-full-data-set/.
26 As cited in Ducharme, "COLUMNS Latest changes to Condominium Act are significant," https://www.fosters.com/story/business/columns/2018/09/02/latest-changes-to-condominium-act-are-significant/10864840007/.
27 Britannica ProCon.org, "FDA-Approved Prescription Drugs Later Pulled from the Market," https://prescriptiondrugs.procon.org/fda-approved-prescription-drugs-later-pulled-from-the-market/.
28 Abramson and Starfield, "The Effect of Conflict of Interest on Biomedical Research and Clinical Practice Guidelines: Can We Trust the Evidence in Evidence-Based Medicine?" https://www.jabfm.org/content/jabfp/18/5/414.full.pdf.
29 MES Truth, "2009 HIV/AIDS Documentary: House of Numbers – Anatomy of an Epidemic," https://www.youtube.com/watch?v=lvDqjXTByF4.
30 Gøtzcshe, *Deadly Medicines and Organized Crime*, 26.
31 Brownstein, "Google Is Burying Alternative Health Sites to Protect People from 'Dangerous' Medical Advice," https://fee.org/articles/google-is-burying-alternative-health-sites-to-protect-people-from-dangerous-medical-advice/.
32 This general point about intentions has been made by Dennis Prager, a political commentator. For more on this topic, see my book *An End to the Upside Down Reset*.
33 Housatonic.Live, "Ep 200.1: Dr. Mark Bailey (author of "A Farewell to Virology") questions pathogenic viruses," https://odysee.com/@Housatonic:0/539-ep-200-1:3.
34 Dr. Sam Bailey, "Death Shot Doctors Stand Down," https://odysee.com/@drsambailey:c/Death-Shot-Doctors-Stand-Down:3?src=embed.
35 Gøtzcshe, *Deadly Medicines and Organized Crime*, 70, 71, 74.
36 Authors Dawn Lester and David Parker often use this analogy, for instance, in their book *What Really Makes You Ill?*, 85.
37 Passon, "Kelvin's Clouds," https://pubs.aip.org/aapt/ajp/article-abstract/89/11/1037/859801/Kelvin-s-clouds?redirectedFrom=fulltext.

I originally heard this mentioned by Dr. Dean Radin. Also see Greene, *The Fabric of the Cosmos*, 9.

38 This analogy has been used by many thinkers. For instance, Dr. Bernardo Kastrup has used it, in addition to Dr. Samantha Bailey and others.

39 Dangor, "CDC's Six-Foot Social Distancing Rule Was 'Arbitrary,' Says Former FDA Commissioner," https://www.forbes.com/sites/graisondangor/2021/09/19/cdcs-six-foot-social-distancing-rule-was-arbitrary-says-former-fda-commissioner/?sh=331efc39e8e6.

40 O'Neill, "Fauci says attacks on him are 'attacks on science,'" https://nypost.com/2021/06/09/fauci-says-attacks-on-him-are-attacks-on-science/.

41 Perry, "Michael Crichton Explains Why There Is 'No Such Thing as Consensus Science,'" https://www.aei.org/carpe-diem/michael-crichton-explains-why-there-is-no-such-thing-as-consensus-science/.

CHAPTER 1: HIV/AIDS

1 World Health Organization, "HIV and AIDS," https://www.who.int/news-room/fact-sheets/detail/hiv-aids.

2 Ibid.

3 Shenton, *Positively False*, lxxxviii.

4 Farber, *Serious Adverse Events*, 1–2.

5 As cited in Banks, *AIDS, Opium, Diamonds, and Empire*, 10. Also see the letter sent to both the editor-in-chief and CEO of *Science* by a number of reputable individuals, dated December 1, 2008. Link to the letter: https://garynull.com/wp-content/uploads/2023/08/081201-Letter-To-Science-Gallo-Papers.pdf.

6 Ibid (in reference to both Banks and the letter to *Science*). The letter to *Science* also includes the following: "In another letter by Gallo, dated one day before he submitted his papers to *Science*, Gallo states, 'It's extremely rare to find fresh cells [from AIDS patients] expressing the virus...cell culture seems to be necessary to induce virus,' a statement which raises the possibility he was working with a laboratory artifact."

7 Ledford, "Luc Montagnier (1932–2022)," https://www.nature.com/articles/d41586-022-00653-y.

8 Farber, *Serious Adverse Events*, xv.

9 Ibid., 13.

10 Duesberg, *Inventing the AIDS Virus*, 4.

11 Banks, *AIDS, Opium, Diamonds, and Empire*, 4.

12 Engelbrecht et al., *Virus Mania*, 103.

13 Mullis, *Dancing Naked in the Mind Field*, 180.

14 Ibid., 171–74.

15 Ibid., 175–77.

16 Shenton, *Positively False*, 151.

17 Farber, *Serious Adverse Events*, 62.

18 Shenton, *Positively False*, 136–37.

19 Ibid., 137.
20 Ibid., 138.
21 Ibid., 142.
22 Banks, *AIDS, Opium, Diamonds, and Empire*, 300.
23 Eduardo Corrochio, "Kary Mullis Explains the PCR Test," https://www.youtube.com/watch?v=ZmZft4fXhQQ.
24 Shenton, *Positively False*, 207–08.
25 Ibid., 208.
26 Ibid., 211.
27 Kennedy Jr., *The Real Anthony Fauci*, 222.
28 Duesberg, *Inventing the AIDS Virus*, 148.
29 Kennedy Jr., *The Real Anthony Fauci*, 223.
30 Engelbrecht et al., *Virus Mania*, 118.
31 Ibid.
32 Ibid., 130.
33 Ibid., 132.
34 Zane, "How the Real-Life Rock Hudson From Hollywood Changed the AIDS Movement," https://www.menshealth.com/entertainment/a32228064/rock-hudson-aids/.
35 Ibid.
36 Engelbrecht, *Virus Mania*, 450–52.
37 Ibid., 151.
38 Hezakya Newz & Films, "1988 THROWBACK: 'DR FAUCI SAYS AZT AIDS DRUG IS SAFE AND EFFECTIVE,'" https://www.youtube.com/watch?v=fKWwEkBZjhM.
39 Engelbrecht, *Virus Mania*, 153.
40 Duesberg, *Inventing the AIDS Virus*, 313.
41 Engelbrecht, *Virus Mania*, 153.
42 As cited in Farber, *Serious Adverse Events*, 68.
43 Engelbrecht, *Virus Mania*, 150.
44 Ibid., 153.
45 Farber, *Serious Adverse Events*, 65.
46 Banks, *AIDS, Opium, Diamonds, and Empire*, 258.
47 Duesberg, *Inventing the AIDS Virus*, 357. Deusberg writes: "But just as soon as Ashe received his AIDS diagnosis in 1988, his doctor pushed him into taking AZT. He started on an unbelievably high dose, nearly double the seriously toxic levels used in the Phase II trial. His doctor only gradually lowered the dose over the next four years. 'I refuse to dwell on how much damage I may have done to myself taking the higher dosage,' Ashe later admitted."
48 More on Arthur Ashe and Magic Johnson in Engelbrecht, *Virus Mania*, 158–61.
49 Duesberg, *Inventing the AIDS Virus*, 340–41.
50 Shenton, *Positively False*, 214.
51 Engelbrecht, *Virus Mania*, 154.
52 Ibid., 145.

53 Ibid., 144.
54 Ibid., 146.
55 Padian et al., "Heterosexual Transmission of Human Immunodeficiency Virus (HIV) in Northern California: Results from a Ten-Year Study," https://academic.oup.com/aje/article/146/4/350/60711?login=false.
56 Banks, *AIDS, Opium, Diamonds, and Empire*, 289.
57 Rasnick, "Rapid Response: Sex has nothing to do with AIDS," https://www.bmj.com/rapid-response/2011/10/29/sex-has-nothing-do-aids. For instance, Dr. Rasnick writes in the letter: "I challenge Dr. Gareth Lloyd to come up with the names (even one will do) of the persons who are documented to have shown that AIDS (or even HIV) is sexually transmitted. I know of no such study. In fact, the scientific, medical literature is full of evidence that neither AIDS nor HIV is sexually transmitted. It is only assumed that they are. The results of the world's best scientific study that attempted to measure the efficiency of heterosexual transmission of antibodies to HIV was conducted by Nancy Padian and her colleagues.... The most striking result of the ten-year study is that Padian et al. did not observe any HIV-negative sex partners becoming HIV-positive from years of unprotected sexual intercourse with their HIV-positive partners. I repeat—NOT ONE HIV-negative sex partner became positive during the 10-year study. Therefore, the observed transmission efficiency was ZERO. However, to avoid reporting a zero efficiency for the sexual transmission of HIV, Padian and colleagues assumed that the HIV-positive sex partners in their study must have become positive through sexual intercourse before entering the study. Using that assumption, they estimated that an HIV-negative woman would have to have sexual intercourse 1,000 times with HIV-positive men before becoming HIV-positive herself. Even more astounding, HIV-negative men would have to have 8,000 sexual contacts before becoming HIV-positive....[There] are additional examples in the literature that neither AIDS nor HIV is sexually transmitted. None of the husbands of HIV-positive women became antibody-positive to HIV over a three-year period."
58 AIDSTruth, "HIV heterosexual transmission and the "Padian paper myth," https://aidstruth.org/misuse-of-studies/padian/.
59 Shenton, *Positively False*, 212.
60 Ibid.
61 Ibid.
62 Question Everything, "Dr Robert Willner Injects 'HIV' into himself on TV," https://www.youtube.com/watch?v=tQCKb1JV-4A.
63 Duesberg, *Inventing the AIDS Virus*, 291–92.
64 Shenton, *Positively False*, 219.
65 Banks, *AIDS, Opium, Diamonds, and Empire*, 5.
66 Ibid., 15.
67 Kennedy Jr., *The Real Anthony Fauci*, 172.

CHAPTER 2: VIRUS ISOLATION

1 See "Read Neville Hodgkinson's summary for the existence of HIV" at http://www.theperthgroup.com/.
2 Dr. Lanka is mentioned in Shenton, *Positively False*, 206–07. His website is in the German language but can be translated into English: https://wissenschafftplus.de/cms/de/empfehlungen.
3 Dr. Tom Cowan, "MY DISCUSSION WITH STEFAN LANKA ABOUT VIROLOGY," https://www.bitchute.com/video/oBJOwK-pgtDqX/. Also see Dr. Lanka's paper titled, "The Misconception called 'Virus,'" https://archive.org/details/paper-virus-lanka-002/mode/2up.
4 Shenton, *Positively False*, 206–07. Also see Dr. Tom Cowan, "MY DISCUSSION WITH STEFAN LANKA ABOUT VIROLOGY," https://www.bitchute.com/video/oBJOwKpgtDqX/.
5 Banks, *AIDS, Opium, Diamonds, and Empire*, 298.
6 Ibid.
7 As cited in Shenton, *Positively False*, 207.
8 Bauer, in the foreword of Shenton, *Positively False*, xvii.
9 As cited in Bailey, "A Farewell to Virology," 22. Also see Bailey, "Fact-check: New Zealand can't find the SARS-CoV-2 virus," https://drsambailey.com/fact-check-new-zealand-cant-find-the-sars-cov-2-virus/.
10 ESR, "Official Information Act Request: FOIA: SARS-COV-2 Proof of Existence," https://www.fluoridefreepeel.ca/wp-content/uploads/2022/08/NZ-ESR-No-Proof-Of-Existence.pdf.
11 As cited in Bailey, "A Farewell to Virology," 22. Also see Bailey, "Fact-check: New Zealand can't find the SARS-CoV-2 virus," https://drsambailey.com/fact-check-new-zealand-cant-find-the-sars-cov-2-virus/.
12 ESR, "Official Information Act Request: SARS-COV-2 Proof of Causation," https://www.fluoridefreepeel.ca/wp-content/uploads/2022/09/2022-08-29-ESR-SARS-COV-2-Proof-of-Causation-Redacted.pdf.
13 Department of Health and Human Services, FOI response: November 2, 2020, https://www.fluoridefreepeel.ca/wp-content/uploads/2020/11/USA-CDC-Virus-Isolation-Response-Scrubbed.pdf.
14 As noted by Dr. Mark Bailey in personal correspondence with the author on September 30, 2023: "Most of us would say that 'COVID-19' is not a specific disease. It has been defined by molecular detection assays, so although there are 'cases,' they are meaningless, as the tests are not clinically validated." See: https://drsambailey.com/the-covid-19-fraud-war-on-humanity/ ("THE THIRD PILLAR: PCR") and https://drsambailey.com/resources/videos/covid-19/what-is-a-covid-19-case/ + https://drsambailey.com/resources/videos/interviews/pcr-pandemic-interview-with-dr-claus-kohnlein/.

15 This question, and some of the subsequent hypotheses discussed, are also explored in greater detail in "The End of COVID" series: https://theendofcovid.com/.

16 As stated in the more-than-600-page book, *A Handbook of Environmental Toxicology (*edited by J.P.F. D'Mello): *Human Disorders and Ecotoxicology* (2020): "It is all too easy to dismiss evidence linking environmental contaminants to ill health in humans....However, several authors contributing to this *Handbook* are at pains to point to biologically plausible mechanisms underlying the said adverse effects." The quotation is from page xxx. Also see, for example, Seneff, *Toxic Legacy: How the Weedkiller Glyphosate Is Destroying Our Health and the Environment;* Connett et al., *The Cause Against Fluoride*; Bryson, *The Fluoride Deception*; and Wicker, *To Dye For: How Toxic Fashion Is Making Us Sick—and How We Can Fight Back.*

17 For example, see Burdick, "4 Studies Add to Evidence of Wireless Technology-Related Electromagnetic Radiation in Humans," https://childrenshealthdefense.org/defender/wireless-technology-electromagnetic-radiation-humans/. Another example is Mercola, "EMF Pollution and Chronic Disease — What's the Connection?" https://childrenshealthdefense.org/defender/emf-pollution-chronic-disease-cola/.

18 For example, see Arthur Firstenberg's *The Invisible Rainbow.*

19 For example, see documents in Balthazar, *Project MK-ULTRA and Mind Control Technology.*

20 Ross, *The CIA Doctors*, 22–23.

21 Tran, "The White House Admits It: We Might Need to Block the Sun to Stop Climate Change," https://news.yahoo.com/white-house-admits-might-block-094049223.html.

22 Bown, *Scurvy*, 3.

23 Crosta, "Everything you need to know about scurvy," https://www.medicalnewstoday.com/articles/155758.

24 Britannica, "Beriberi," https://www.britannica.com/science/beriberi. Also see Engelbrecht et al., *Virus Mania*, 65–66.

25 Britannica, "Pellagra," https://www.britannica.com/science/pellagra. Also see Engelbrecht et al., *Virus Mania*, 65–66.

26 Hammond, "Cowan and Haberland Illuminate the Dogma of Virus Denialism," https://www.jeremyrhammond.com/2022/11/09/study-finds-42-false-discovery-rate-for-sars-cov-2-pcr-tests/.

27 WISN, "'Dying of' vs. 'dying with': Medical Examiner explains COVID-19 difference," https://www.wisn.com/article/covid-19-dying-of-vs-dying-with-medical-examiner-explains-difference/34909031.

28 Manek, "Do women's periods really sync up?" https://www.sciencefocus.com/the-human-body/do-periods-sync.

29 Many holistic practitioners use language like this, but it's also mentioned explicitly in Lester and Parker, *What Really Makes You Ill?*, 686.

30 Grafe, *A History of Experimental Virology*, 3–5.

31 Dr. Sam Bailey, "Gain Of Function Garbage," https://drsambailey.com/resources/videos/covid-19/gain-of-function-garbage//. Also see Dr. Sam Bailey, "Gain Of Function Gaslighting," https://drsambailey.com/resources/videos/covid-19/gain-of-function-gaslighting/.

32 I participated in this event as an interviewee for three segments that related to my books *An End to the Upside Down Reset* and *An End to Upside Down Liberty*. At the time of my participation, I was aware of the No Virus debate but had not studied the arguments.

33 For more information on the split within the health-freedom community, see Dr. Sam Bailey, "'Viruses' – Baileys, Cowan & Kaufman Respond To Del Bigtree," https://odysee.com/@drsambailey:c/Viruses-Baileys-Cowan-Kaufman-Respond-To-Del-Bigtree:b. Also see Dr. Sam Bailey, "The Follies of Peter McCullough," https://odysee.com/@drsambailey:c/The-Follies-of-Peter-McCullough:4; TheWayFwrd, "OUR RESPONSE TO JJ COUEY," https://www.bitchute.com/video/iZJAZEkra4uI/, which features Dr. Thomas Cowan, Dr. Andrew Kaufman, Dr. Mark Bailey, Christine Massey, and Alec Zeck; and EarthNewspaper.com, "ANTIVIRAL OR NONSENSE BY DR. THOMAS COWAN," https://www.bitchute.com/video/5NtlfxqCBzw7/.

34 For instance, see Cowan, *Breaking the Spell*, 27. He challenges the belief in cellular structures such as ribosomes: "Since the early discovery of ribosomes, they have been seen only using the high magnification of the electron microscope. They are always seen as perfect circles, either attached to the snake-like structure called the 'endoplasmic reticulum' or floating free in the cytoplasm (the watery part of the cell outside the nucleus). However, we must realize that any structure that is always perfectly circular in a two-dimensional image must have been spherical in three-dimensional 'life.' To find a ribosome, the homogenization of the cell is required, meaning that it's put into a kind of blender. When any structure that is perfectly spherical is put into a blender, it's impossible that it would be cut into perfect circles. This defies the basic laws of spherical geometry. In other words, the perfect circles seen on electron micrograph images for decades—drawn in all modern images of the cell—must be artifacts. That ribosomes can't possibly exist inside an intact cell is the conclusion reached by [Harold] Hillman, who discussed the history of ribosomes in many of his books and showed, step by step, that no one has ever proven that such a structure actually exists inside the cell. The circles are likely stained gas bubbles that are the inevitable result of how the tissue is prepared. Let's look at another structure seen in all drawings of the components of a human cell. The endoplasmic reticulum is the long tube-like structure that, in

these drawings, is attached to the lining of the nucleus and to the cell wall. Like ribosomes, the endoplasmic reticulum is seen only using an electron micrograph, and, again like ribosomes, it is a structure crucial to the modern understanding of how a cell functions. It was 'invented' to solve the problem biologists faced when they theorized that the DNA is contained in the nucleus, which is bound by a membrane." Also see Dr. Tom Cowan, "NUCLEAR ATOM & RESPONSE TO VERNON COLEMAN – 9/6/23 WEBINAR," https://www.bitchute.com/video/BC25ikU2sTKt/. The general principles of questioning assumptions of biology are shown here: https://drtomcowan.com/pages/the-new-biology.

35 For example, see TheWayFwrd, "OUR RESPONSE TO JJ COUEY," https://www.bitchute.com/video/iZJAZEkra4uI/, which features Dr. Thomas Cowan, Dr. Andrew Kaufman, Dr. Mark Bailey, Christine Massey, and Alec Zeck.

36 For example, see "Alec Zeck | C.A.U.S.E Fest Nashville 2023," https://rumble.com/v35zsqe-alec-zeck-c.a.u.s.e-fest-nashville-2023.html.

37 *Merriam-Webster*, "isolate," https://www.merriam-webster.com/dictionary/isolate.

38 Dr. Montagnier's response was specifically regarding the purpose of purifying a virus. houseofnumbers, "Prof. Luc Montagnier's Extended House of Numbers Interview," https://www.youtube.com/watch?v=PyPq-waF-h4.

39 For example, see TheWayFwrd, "OUR RESPONSE TO JJ COUEY," https://www.bitchute.com/video/iZJAZEkra4uI/, which features Dr. Thomas Cowan, Dr. Andrew Kaufman, Dr. Mark Bailey, Christine Massey, and Alec Zeck.

40 Cowan, *Breaking the Spell*, 1.

41 Broad Institute, "David Baltimore, Ph.D.," https://www.broadinstitute.org/bios/david-baltimore.

42 MES Truth, "2009 HIV/AIDS Documentary: House of Numbers – Anatomy of an Epidemic," https://www.youtube.com/watch?v=lvDqjXTByF4.

43 Grafe, *A History of Experimental Virology*, 4–5.

44 McBean, *The Poisoned Needle*, chapter 10 ("What Is a Virus?").

45 Dr. Tom Cowan, "MY DISCUSSION WITH STEFAN LANKA ABOUT VIROLOGY," https://www.bitchute.com/video/oBJOwKpgtDqX/.

46 The Nobel Prize, "The Nobel Prize in Physiology or Medicine 1969," https://www.nobelprize.org/prizes/medicine/1969/summary/.

47 This point has been made by Dr. Andrew Kaufman, for example, in personal correspondence with the author on October 2, 2023. Dr. Kaufman notes that a pure bacterial culture in which bacteriophages are found represents a stressful situation for bacteria: typically, they exist in more diverse environments. Bacteriophages could thus be viewed almost like spores that are part of the process of a bacteria's resistance to

the situation. Similarly, Dr. Kaufman notes that so-called giant viruses that allegedly "infect" sea algae might actually be helping the algae survive. Virologist Dr. Stefan Lanka remarks, "As a young student, I myself isolated such a 'phage' structure from a sea algae, and believed at that time to have discovered the first harmless virus, the first stable "virus host system." See Lanka, "The Misconception called 'Virus,'" https://archive.org/details/paper-virus-lanka-002/mode/2up.

48 NIH, "The Discovery of the Double Helix, 1951-1953," https://profiles.nlm.nih.gov/spotlight/sc/feature/doublehelix.

49 Lanka, "The Misconception called 'Virus,'" https://archive.org/details/paper-virus-lanka-002/mode/2up.

50 Dr. Sam Bailey, "Settling The Virus Debate" Statement," https://drsambailey.com/resources/settling-the-virus-debate/.

51 Ravindran et al., "A Non-enveloped Virus Hijacks Host Disaggregation Machinery to Translocate across the Endoplasmic Reticulum Membrane," https://journals.plos.org/plospathogens/article?id=10.1371/journal.ppat.1005086.

52 As cited in Engelbrecht et al., *Virus Mania*, 66–67.

53 Morgan, "The Physician Who Presaged the Germ Theory of Disease Nearly 500 Years Ago," https://www.scientificamerican.com/article/the-physician-who-presaged-the-germ-theory-of-disease-nearly-500-years-ago/.

54 Britannica, "History of optical microscopes," https://www.britannica.com/technology/microscope/History-of-optical-microscopes. Britannica, "Antonie van Leeuwenhoek," https://www.britannica.com/biography/Antonie-van-Leeuwenhoek.

55 Britannica, "Vaccine development of Louis Pasteur," https://www.britannica.com/biography/Louis-Pasteur/Vaccine-development.

56 Britannica, "Louis Pasteur," https://www.britannica.com/biography/Louis-Pasteur.

57 Geison, *The Private Science of Louis Pasteur*, 9–10.

58 Roingeard, "Viral detection by electron microscopy: past, present and future," https://www.ncbi.nlm.nih.gov/pmc/articles/PMC7161876/.

59 Ibid.

60 As stated in the textbook *Virology* by Carter and Saunders (p. 4): "Evidence of the existence of very small infectious agents was first provided in the late nineteenth century by two scientists working independently: Martinus Beijerinck in Holland and Dimitri Ivanovski in Russia. They made extracts from diseased plants, which we now know were infected with tobacco mosaic virus, and passed the extracts through fine filters. The filtrates contained an agent that was able to infect new plants, but no bacteria could be cultured from the filtrates. The agent remained infective through several transfers to new plants, eliminating the possibility of a toxin. Beijerinck called the agent a 'virus,' and the term has been in use ever since." Note that this textbook assumes that a virus was there even though at the time of the

experiment it was not visible. Also, the authors do not raise the environmental factors that impacted the plants, as pointed out in Bailey, "A Farewell to Virology," 15, https://drsambailey.com/a-farewell-to-virology-expert-edition/.

61 Bailey, "A Farewell to Virology," 15, https://drsambailey.com/a-farewell-to-virology-expert-edition/.

62 For a discussion of Tobacco Mosaic Virus, see Ibid., 15–16.

63 For more on Tobacco mosaic virus, see Dr. Sam Bailey, "Tobacco Mosaic "Virus" – The beginning & end of virology," https://drsambailey.com/resources/videos/viruses-unplugged/tobacco-mosaic-virus-the-beginning-and-end-of-virology/.

64 Wikipedia, "Tobacco mosaic virus," https://en.wikipedia.org/wiki/Tobacco_mosaic_virus. Accessed on September 20, 2023.

65 Bailey, "A Farewell to Virology," 16–17, https://drsambailey.com/a-farewell-to-virology-expert-edition/.

66 Dr. Tom Cowan, "MY DISCUSSION WITH STEFAN LANKA ABOUT VIROLOGY," https://www.bitchute.com/video/oBJOwKpgtDqX/.

67 In general, the fluids may be put through a centrifuge, and only a fraction of the result moves onto the next step. The No Virus group has often critiqued this method, because even after separating some of the fluids with a centrifuge, there needs to be a way to show that *only* the virus is contained in the separated portion—and not other cellular material from the sample that could alter the experiment's results.

68 Dr. Tom Cowan, "MY DISCUSSION WITH STEFAN LANKA ABOUT VIROLOGY," https://www.bitchute.com/video/oBJOwKpgtDqX/.

69 For more on the fundamental arguments by the No Virus camp, see the following presentation by Alec Zeck, Jordan Grant, MD, Jacob Diaz, and Mike Donio at https://unite.live/the-way-forward/the-way-forward?recording_id=1110.

70 Cowan, *Breaking the Spell*, 6–8.

71 Enders and Peebles, "Propagation in Tissue Cultures of Cytopathogenic Agents from Patients with Measles," 11.

72 Ibid.

73 As noted in Dr. Bailey's personal correspondence with the author on September 30, 2023.

74 See Bailey, "A Farewell to Virology," 17–18. Also, Drs. Cowan and Kaufman (among others) have pointed to a line in the 1954 Enders and Peebles paper that they feel is suggestive that they performed an additional, telling experiment, but they didn't describe it in detail. The researchers found cellular breakdown in an uninoculated culture of monkey kidney cells that "could not be distinguished with confidence from the viruses obtained from measles." In other words, when the human fluids were not added to the culture, the same cellular breakdown occurred. This has been interpreted to mean that something in

the "soup" itself caused cells to break down, not an alleged virus. As is the case with many technical papers, there are varying interpretations, and one allegation against the No Virus position here is that it takes the line out of context. However, Dr. Cowan points to an additional line from a 1957 follow-up paper by Dr. Enders, in which Dr. Enders cites another virologist who said that a particle was found that was "indistinguishable" from the virus. For more on these studies, see Cowan, *Breaking the Spell*, 7; Enders and Peebles, "Propagation in Tissue Cultures of Cytopathogenic Agents from Patients with Measles," 15. Also see DrAndrewKaufman, "Virus-Isolation Is It Real? Andrew_Kaufman Responds To Jeremy Hammond," https://odysee.com/@DrAndrewKaufman:f/Virus_Isolation_Is_It_Real_Andrew_Kaufman_Responds_To_Jeremy-Hammond:9.

75 Bailey, "A Farewell to Virology," 18, https://drsambailey.com/a-farewell-to-virology-expert-edition/.

76 DrAndrewKaufman, "Virus-Isolation: Is It Real? Andrew_Kaufman Responds To Jeremy Hammond," https://odysee.com/@DrAndrewKaufman:f/Virus_Isolation_Is_It_Real_Andrew_Kaufman_Responds_To_Jeremy-Hammond:9.

77 *Nature*, submission guidelines," https://www.nature.com/srep/author-instructions/submission-guidelines#methods. Dr. Kaufman pointed this out to the author in personal correspondence on October 2, 2023.

78 Here, I am summarizing the perspective held by many members of the No Virus camp. Many of them cite the work of Harold Hillman, PhD, who questioned the fundamentals of cell biology. For example, see his work titled *The Case for New Paradigms in Cell Biology and Neurobiology* (among others).

79 Dr. Sam Bailey, "Electron Microscopy and Unidentified 'Viral' Objects," https://drsambailey.com/resources/videos/covid-19/electron-microscopy-and-unidentified-viral-objects/.

80 Ibid.

81 Harold Hillman, PhD, made arguments like this that caused him to challenge cell biology more broadly. For example, see his work titled *The Case for New Paradigms in Cell Biology and Neurobiology* (among others).

82 Dr. Sam Bailey, "Electron Microscopy and Unidentified 'Viral' Objects," https://drsambailey.com/resources/videos/covid-19/electron-microscopy-and-unidentified-viral-objects/.

83 Science Learning Hub, "Preparing samples for the electron microscope," https://www.sciencelearn.org.nz/resources/500-preparing-samples-for-the-electron-microscope.

84 Microscope Master, "What is Cryo-Electron Microscopy?" https://www.microscopemaster.com/cryo-electron-microscopy.html. Also see Carter and Saunders, *Virology*, 16: "Cryo-electron microscopy techniques are more recent. For these techniques, wet specimens are rapidly cooled to a temperature below -160 degrees C, freezing the water

as a glass-like material. The images are recorded while the specimen is frozen."

85 Bullock et al., "Difficulties in Differentiating Coronaviruses from Subcellular Structures in Human Tissues by Electron Microscopy," https://wwwnc.cdc.gov/eid/article/27/4/20-4337_article.

86 Dr. Sam Bailey, "Electron Microscopy and Unidentified 'Viral' Objects," https://drsambailey.com/resources/videos/covid-19/electron-microscopy-and-unidentified-viral-objects/.

87 As noted by Dr. Mark Bailey, a "common cold unit" was set up in the United Kingdom after World War II. He comments, "What was interesting is that after four decades, they basically had nothing that your grandma couldn't tell you about the common cold." See TrainofThoughts, "Maajid Nawaz – Mark Bailey – Why The Covid Virus Has Never Been Isolated – Jan 08 2023," https://rumble.com/v25m25v-maajid-nawaz-mark-bailey-why-the-covid-virus-has-never-been-isolated-jan-08.html.

88 Dr. Sam Bailey, "Electron Microscopy and Unidentified 'Viral' Objects," https://drsambailey.com/resources/videos/covid-19/electron-microscopy-and-unidentified-viral-objects/. Almeida and Tyrrell, "The Morphology of Three Previously Uncharacterized Human Respiratory Viruses that Grow in Organ Culture," https://www.microbiologyresearch.org/content/journal/jgv/10.1099/0022-1317-1-2-175.

89 The 1967 paper discussed *claims* to have done a control (though it provides minimal detail), but because the virus wasn't isolated, conducting a proper control was not possible. See Almeida and Tyrrell, "The Morphology of Three Previously Uncharacterized Human Respiratory Viruses That Grow in Organ Culture." The paper states: "Virus particles or viral components were detected in almost all the cultures inoculated with known viruses, and in no instance in an uninoculated control. An additional control was provided by examining cultures that had been inoculated with herpes simplex and vaccinia viruses and then not incubated but held at 4°. No virus particles were seen in these preparations." However, since the virus was not isolated, the researchers couldn't have concluded that what they saw were viruses. The images could have simply been capturing other cellular material of unknown origin. Furthermore, the study didn't demonstrate that the thing seen under the microscope was a replication-competent intracellular parasite. The particle wasn't seen performing all of those steps.

90 Dr. Sam Bailey, "Stefan Lanka: 'Virus, It's Time To Go,'" https://odysee.com/@drsambailey:c/Stefan-Lanka-Virus-Its-Time-To-Go:1?src=embed.

91 Dr. Tom Cowan, "MY DISCUSSION WITH STEFAN LANKA ABOUT VIROLOGY," https://www.bitchute.com/video/oBJOwKpgtDqX/.

92 Ibid.

93 For example, for a discussion of spike proteins, see Dr. Sam Bailey, "Peter McCullough's Shedding Stories," https://drsambailey.com/resources/videos/vaccines/peter-mcculloughs-shedding-stories/.
94 Bailey, "A Farewell to Virology," 28.
95 Ibid., 31.
96 Personal correspondence with Dr. Andrew Kaufman on October 2, 2023. Also see Dr. Tom Cowan, "Discussing the actual origin of the lab leak theory- Webinar from 10/18/23," https://rumble.com/v3q956g-discussing-the-actual-origin-of-the-lab-leak-theory-webinar-from-101823.html?mref=6zof&mc=dgip3&ep=2.
97 Bailey, "A Farewell to Virology," 30.
98 Ibid., 34.
99 Personal correspondence with Dr. Andrew Kaufman on October 2, 2023.
100 "A Farewell to Virology" is available at https://drsambailey.com/a-farewell-to-virology-expert-edition/. Also see Drs. Mark Bailey and Thomas Cowan's October 11, 2023 webinar, which discusses the HART Group's discussion about the No Virus position—including a discussion about genetic sequencing: Dr.TomCowan, WEBINAR WITH DR. MARK BAILEY ON THE HART GROUP: OCTOBER 11, 2023, https://www.bitchute.com/video/lAJp8FwPrMSi/.
101 The Tom Woods Show, "Ep. 2282 Do Viruses Exist?" https://tomwoods.com/ep-2282-do-viruses-exist/#disqus_thread.
102 As noted by Dr. Mark Bailey in personal correspondence with the author on October 7, 2023. The ivermectin study referenced is Caley et al., "The FDA-approved drug ivermectin inhibits the replication of SARS-CoV-2 in vitro," https://doi.org/10.1016/j.antiviral.2020.104787.
103 Cowan, *Breaking the Spell*, 4. In personal correspondence with Dr. Kaufman on October 2, 2023, he clarified an error in Dr. Cowan's quotation: it was Dr. Kaufman, rather than Dr. Cowan, who asked the scientists. This clarification is reflected in brackets within the quotation.
104 Banks, *AIDS, Opium, Diamonds, and Empire*, 298.
105 Cowan, *Breaking the Spell*, 5.
106 DrAndrewKaufman, "VIRUS-ISOLATION IS IT REAL? ANDREW KAUFMAN MD RESPONDS TO JEREMY HAMMOND," https://www.bitchute.com/video/UnpfmjmXNH0O/. He cites "Purification of Bacteriophages Using Anion-Exchange Chromatography," https://pubmed.ncbi.nlm.nih.gov/29134587/. "Standardized bacteriophage purification for personalized phage therapy," https://www.nature.com/articles/s41596-020-0346-0. In personal correspondence with the author on October 2, 2023, Dr. Kaufman also referenced papers showing methods of isolating exosomes: Patel et al., "Comparative analysis of exosome isolation methods using culture supernatant for optimum yield, purity and downstream applications," https://www.nature.com/articles/s41598-019-41800-2; Chen

et al., "Review on Strategies and Technologies for Exosome Isolation and Purification," https://www.frontiersin.org/articles/10.3389/fbioe.2021.811971; and Rai et al., "A Protocol for Isolation, Purification, Characterization, and Functional Dissection of Exosomes," https://pubmed.ncbi.nlm.nih.gov/33420988/.

107 Dr. Sam Bailey, "Stefan Lanka: 'Virus, It's Time To Go,'" https://odysee.com/@drsambailey:c/Stefan-Lanka-Virus-Its-Time-To-Go:1?src=embed. Dr. Lanka also writes: "The (bacterio)phages have indeed been isolated in the meaning of the word 'isolation' with standard methods (density gradient centrifugation). Immediately after the isolation they have been photographed in an electron microscope, their purity is determined and then their components, their proteins and their DNA have been biochemically described all at once, in one single paper....With respect to all 'viruses' of humans, animals or plants, however, no virus was ever isolated, photographed in an isolated form and its components were never biochemically characterised all at once, from the 'isolate.' In reality, there was a consensus process, taking place over quite a number of years, in which single particles of dead cells were theoretically ascribed to a totally virtual virus model. The phages served as a model for this entire interpretation process, as we can see clearly from the first drawings of a 'virus.'" See Lanka, "The Misconception called 'Virus,'" https://archive.org/details/paper-virus-lanka-002/mode/2up.

108 The HART Group's October 4, 2023, article, "Why HART uses the virus model" can be accessed at: https://www.hartgroup.org/virus-model/. For a point-by-point rebuttal of the HART Group's contentions, see Dr.TomCowan, "WEBINAR WITH DR. MARK BAILEY ON THE HART GROUP: OCTOBER 11, 2023, https://www.bitchute.com/video/lAJp8FwPrMSi/.

109 Cowan, *Breaking the Spell*, 13.

110 Ibid., 14.

111 For example, as mentioned in a previous endnote, Drs. Cowan and Kaufman (among others) have pointed to a line in the 1954 Enders and Peebles paper that they feel is suggestive that they performed an additional, telling experiment, but they didn't describe it in detail. The researchers found cellular breakdown in an uninoculated culture of monkey kidney cells that "could not be distinguished with confidence from the viruses obtained from measles." In other words, when the human fluids were not added to the culture, the same cellular breakdown occurred. This has been interpreted to mean that something in the "soup" itself causes cells to break down, not an alleged virus. As is the case with many technical papers, there are varying interpretations, and one allegation against the No Virus position here is that it takes the line out of context. However, Dr. Cowan points to an additional line from a 1957 follow-up paper by Dr. Enders, in which Dr. Enders cites another virologist who said that a particle was

found that was "indistinguishable" from the virus. For more on these studies, see Cowan, *Breaking the Spell*, 7; Enders and Peebles, "Propagation in Tissue Cultures of Cytopathogenic Agents from Patients with Measles," 15. DrAndrewKaufman, "Virus-Isolation Is It Real? Andrew_Kaufman Responds To Jeremy Hammond," https://odysee.com/@DrAndrewKaufman:f/Virus_Isolation_Is_It_Real_Andrew_Kaufman_Responds_To_Jeremy-Hammond:9. Additionally, in personal correspondence with Dr. Kaufman on October 2, 2023, he referenced an early paper on monkeypox suggesting that the cell-culture methodology itself can cause cells to break down. See von Magnus et al, "A Pox-like Disease in Cynomolgus Monkeys," https://onlinelibrary.wiley.com/doi/10.1111/j.1699-0463.1959.tb00328.x.

112 Dr. Sam Bailey, "The Measles Myth," https://odysee.com/@drsambailey:c/themeaslesmyth:0.

113 Enders and Peebles, "Propagation in tissue cultures of cytopathogenic agents from patients with measles."

114 Bech, "Studies on measles virus in monkey kidney tissue cultures," https://pubmed.ncbi.nlm.nih.gov/13508251/. Some websites state that this paper was published in 1959; however, PubMed shows that it was published in 1958.

115 Nakai and Imagawa, "Electron Microscopy of Measles Virus Replication," https://www.ncbi.nlm.nih.gov/pmc/articles/PMC375751/.

116 Lund et al., "The Molecular Length of Measles Virus RNA and the Structural Organization of Measles Nucleocapsids," https://www.microbiologyresearch.org/content/journal/jgv/10.1099/0022-1317-65-9-1535.

117 Horikami and Moyer, "Structure, transcription, and replication of measles virus," https://pubmed.ncbi.nlm.nih.gov/7789161/.

118 Daikoku et al., "Analysis of Morphology and Infectivity of Measles Virus Particles," Analysis of Morphology and Infectivity of Measles Virus Particles," https://www.semanticscholar.org/paper/Analysis-of-Morphology-and-Infectivity-of-Measles-Eriko-Daikoku/0b85babe55d54b0f58bca35f586852786f25b088.

119 Dr. Sam Bailey, "Stefan Lanka: 'Virus, It's Time To Go,'" https://odysee.com/@drsambailey:c/Stefan-Lanka-Virus-Its-Time-To-Go:1?src=embed.

120 Ibid. Also discussed in Markolin, *Measles Virus Put to the Test*, https://learninggnm.com/SBS/documents/Lanka_Bardens_Trial_E.pdf. Dr. Markolin writes: "According to the minutes of the court proceedings (p. 7/ first paragraph), Andreas Podbielski, head of the Department of Medical Microbiology, Virology and Hygiene at the University Hospital in Rostock, who was one of the appointed experts at the trial, stated that even though the existence of the measles virus could be concluded from the summary of the six papers submitted by Dr. Bardens, none of the authors had conducted any controlled experiments in accordance with internationally defined rules and principles of good

scientific practice (see also the method of 'indirect evidence'). Professor Podbielski considers this lack of control experiments explicitly as a 'methodological weakness' of these publications, which are after all the relevant studies on the subject (there are no other publications trying to attempt to prove the existence of the measles virus). Thus, at this point, a publication about the existence of the measles virus that stands the test of good science has yet to be delivered."

121 Dr. Sam Bailey, "Stefan Lanka: 'Virus, It's Time To Go,'" https://odysee.com/@drsambailey:c/Stefan-Lanka-Virus-Its-Time-To-Go:1?src=embed.

122 Dr. Sam Bailey, "Marvin vs. Virology: COVID Taken to Court," https://odysee.com/@drsambailey:c/Marvin-vs-Virology-COVID-Taken-To-Court:3.

123 Dr. Sam Bailey, "Runaway Virology—Marvin Win in Court," https://odysee.com/@drsambailey:c/Runaway-Virology-Marvin-Wins-In-Court:b?src=embed.

124 ChrisMasseyFOIs, "OFFICIAL EVIDENCE THAT VIROLOGY IS PSEUDOSCIENCE – CHRISTINE MASSEY JUNE 10 2023," https://www.bitchute.com/video/gvu4NbieSuVb/.

125 Department of Health and Human Services, "FOI response: November 2, 2020," https://www.fluoridefreepeel.ca/wp-content/uploads/2020/11/USA-CDC-Virus-Isolation-Response-Scrubbed.pdf.

126 Ibid.

127 Department of Health and Human Services, "FOI response: March 1, 2021," https://www.fluoridefreepeel.ca/wp-content/uploads/2021/03/CDC-March-1-2021-SARS-COV-2-Isolation-Response-Redacted.pdf.

128 UK Health Security Agency, "FOI Response 25 March 2022," https://www.fluoridefreepeel.ca/wp-content/uploads/2022/05/UK-HSA-isolation-sequencing-methods-PACKAGE-redacted.pdf.

129 Public Health Agency of Canada, "Response to Christine Massey 20 December, 2021," https://www.fluoridefreepeel.ca/wp-content/uploads/2022/01/PHAC-ANY-virus-PACKAGE-redacted.pdf.

130 See details of each response at Fluoride Free Peel, "FOIs reveal that health/science institutions have no record of any 'virus' having been found in a host and isolated/purified. Because virology isn't a science," https://www.fluoridefreepeel.ca/fois-reveal-that-health-science-institutions-have-no-record-of-any-virus-having-been-isolated-purified-virology-isnt-a-science/. Massey walks through her website in this video: ChrisMasseyFOIs, "OFFICIAL EVIDENCE THAT VIROLOGY IS PSEUDOSCIENCE – CHRISTINE MASSEY JUNE 10, 2023," https://www.bitchute.com/video/gvu4NbieSuVb/.

131 Bailey, "A Farewell to Virology," 19.

132 Cowan et al., "Settling the Virus Debate," https://drsambailey.com/wp-content/uploads/2022/07/SETTLING-THE-VIRUS-DEBATE-Source.pdf.

133 Dr. Sam Bailey, "Stefan Lanka: 'Virus, It's Time To Go,'" https://odysee.com/@drsambailey:c/Stefan-Lanka-Virus-Its-Time-To-Go:1?src=embed.
134 Official Church of the FSM, https://www.spaghettimonster.org/.

CHAPTER 3: HOW TO DEMONSTRATE THAT A GERM CAUSES DISEASE

1 Bailey, "A Farewell to Virology," 7.
2 Dr. Sam Bailey, "Koch's Postulates: Germ School Dropout," https://drsambailey.com/resources/videos/germ-theory/kochs-postulates-germ-school-dropout/.
3 Ibid. Also see Dr. Sam Bailey, "TB: Cows, Lies & Koch-Ups," https://odysee.com/@drsambailey:c/TB-Cows-Lies-And-Koch-Ups:a.
4 World Health Organization, "Tuberculosis," https://www.who.int/news-room/fact-sheets/detail/tuberculosis.
5 Dr. Sam Bailey, "TB: Cows, Lies & Koch-Ups," https://odysee.com/@drsambailey:c/TB-Cows-Lies-And-Koch-Ups:a.
6 Also, recent papers explicitly discuss Koch's postulates, which suggest that they are indeed still relevant. For example, a 2020 SARS-CoV-2 paper mentions that it does not fulfill Koch's postulates. See Bailey, "A Farewell to Virology," 7, https://drsambailey.com/a-farewell-to-virology-expert-edition/.
7 Mayo Clinic, "E. coli," https://www.mayoclinic.org/diseases-conditions/e-coli/symptoms-causes/syc-20372058.
8 Cleveland Clinic, "Staph Infection," https://my.clevelandclinic.org/health/diseases/21165-staph-infection-staphylococcus-infection.
9 As noted by Dr. Andrew Kaufman in personal correspondence with the author on October 2, 2023, humans are part of nature rather than separate from it. To specify "in nature" creates an artificial divide. However, this framing is included because our society currently has such a bias.
10 According to Dr. Caroline Markolin, in German New Medicine, bacteria are viewed in the following manner: "During the healing process, bacteria help to replenish the tissue loss that took place in the conflict-active phase. Most bacteria are specialized. Staphylococcus bacteria, for example, support the reconstruction of bone tissue; streptococcus bacteria help to rebuild tissue necroses in the ovaries. In PCL-A, bacteria form abscesses. Bacteria also participate in the healing of wounds caused by injuries." German New Medicine is discussed further in chapter 7 of this book and the quotation comes from the following website: https://learninggnm.com/SBS/documents/five_laws.html. These hypotheses warrant further investigation.
11 Britannica, "Endotoxin," https://www.britannica.com/science/endotoxin. Specific toxins listed here were mentioned by Dr. Andrew Kaufman in personal correspondence with the author on October 4, 2023.
12 As noted by Dr. Andrew Kaufman in personal correspondence with the author on October 2, 2023.

13 Dr. Sam Bailey, "TB: Cows, Lies & Koch-Ups," https://odysee.com/@drsambailey:c/TB-Cows-Lies-And-Koch-Ups:a. Many terrain theorists also reference "pleomorphism"—the idea that bacteria can change their form. So perhaps in some instances what we observe under a microscope is a certain form of a bacterium at that time because it's responding to a particular environmental condition. Furthermore, under the theory of pleomorphism, the bacterium can change depending on the environment's demands. More specifically, the fundamental particle, under this theory, is theorized to be a *microzyma* that transforms into a type of bacterium (see the work of Antoine Béchamp). This area of research is important and deserves further attention.

14 Fluoride Free Peel, "Do health and science institutions have studies proving that bacteria CAUSE disease?" https://www.fluoridefreepeel.ca/do-health-authorities-have-studies-proving-that-bacteria-cause-disease-lets-find-out-via-freedom-of-information/.

15 Dr. Sam Bailey, "5 Spectacular Fails From Germ Theory," https://odysee.com/@drsambailey:c/5-Spectacular-Fails-From-Germ-Theory:c?src=embed.

16 Ibid.

17 This point about epidemiological observations has been made by Dr. Thomas Cowan, Dr. Samantha Bailey, and others.

18 Cowan, *The Truth About Contagion*, 3. Also see Dharan and Aarattuthodi, "Rivers's Postulates Fulfilled for Blue Catfish Alloherpesvirus," which includes a summary of Rivers's postulates. The paper claims to have met the postulates, but isolation of the virus is not validated. All the paper says is: "A cell culture viable isolate of BCAHV (S98-675) was received from Dr. Larry Hanson, College of Veterinary Medicine, Mississippi State University." The reader is thus left to guess what was in that "isolate." If it was "isolated" by following the gold-standard method of virology, then it wasn't a true isolation (as discussed in chapter 2). Link to the study: https://sciencepublishinggroup.com/journal/paperinfo?journalid=384&doi=10.11648/j.fem.20210703.12.

19 Cowan, *The Truth About Contagion*, 3.

20 BenGreenfield Life, "Ben's New Dietary Protocol, Vegetables Vs. Viruses, Whether Viruses Really Exist & Much More With Dr. Thomas Cowan," https://bengreenfieldlife.com/podcast/tom-cowan-podcast/.

21 As noted in personal correspondence with Dr. Andrew Kaufman on October 3, 2023, sometimes the full spectrum of symptoms aren't even replicated for the disease that's being studied.

22 TrainofThoughts, "Maajid Nawaz – Mark Bailey – Why The Covid Virus Has Never Been Isolated – Jan 08 2023," https://rumble.com/v25m25v-maajid-nawaz-mark-bailey-why-the-covid-virus-has-never-been-isolated-jan-08.html.

23 Dr. Sam Bailey, "5 Spectacular Fails From Germ Theory," https://odysee.com/@drsambailey:c/5-Spectacular-Fails-From-Germ-Theory:c?src=embed.

24 The ideas expressed here reflect a synthesis of many other thinkers' ideas. For example, see Dr. Sam Bailey, "Germ Theory vs Terrain Theory," https://odysee.com/@drsambailey:c/germ-theory-vs-terrain-theory:0?src=embed&t=348.702826.

25 These points were noted by Dr. Mark Bailey in personal correspondence with the author on October 5, 2023. Also see Dr. Sam Bailey, "The Truth About Antibiotics," https://drsambailey.com/resources/videos/germ-theory/the-truth-about-antibiotics/.

CHAPTER 4: REVISITING INFECTIOUS DISEASES

1 As noted by Dr. Andrew Kaufman in personal correspondence with the author on October 2, 2023, there are some diseases for which the cause is well known. For instance, mesothelioma is often caused by asbestos.

2 Lester and Parker, *What Really Makes You Ill*, 51.

3 CDC, "What is Polio?" https://www.cdc.gov/polio/what-is-polio/index.htm.

4 Lester and Parker, *What Really Makes You Ill*, 54.

5 As emphasized by Dr. Mark Bailey in personal correspondence with the author on October 3, 2023.

6 In fact, Drs. Flexner and Lewis commented that they were unable to "transmit the disease" when they injected animals in their spinal cord or peritoneal cavity, so they then injected monkeys via the brain. See Flexner and Lewis, "The Transmission of Acute Poliomyelitis to Monkeys."

7 For example, see Dr. Tom Cowan, "HOW TO MAKE A POLIO VACCINE + A REBUTTAL – WEBINAR FROM AUGUST 30TH, 2023," https://www.bitchute.com/video/WaPyKutv4Oz9/. Also see the many videos posted by Dr. Samantha Bailey at https://drsambailey.com/.

8 Engdahl, "Toxicology vs Virology: Rockefeller Institute and the Criminal Polio Fraud," http://williamengdahl.com/englishNEO12July2022.php.

9 Listed on Christine Massey's website: https://www.fluoridefreepeel.ca/fois-reveal-that-health-science-institutions-have-no-record-of-any-virus-having-been-isolated-purified-virology-isnt-a-science/.

10 For example, see West, *DDT Polio*, 22.

11 Engelbrecht et al., 79–80.

12 Engdahl, "Toxicology vs Virology: Rockefeller Institute and the Criminal Polio Fraud," http://williamengdahl.com/englishNEO12July2022.php.

13 Ibid.

14 Janssen, "When Polio Triggered Fear and Panic Among Parents in the 1950s," https://www.history.com/news/polio-fear-post-wwii-era.

For more on the use of DDT to try to stop the spread of polio, see Conis, "A misfire in fighting polio provides clues as to how we'll beat covid," https://www.washingtonpost.com/outlook/2022/04/14/misfire-fighting-polio-provides-clues-how-well-beat-covid/. The author writes about "the forgotten story of how Americans once resorted to spraying a now-banned pesticide, DDT, to combat polio is a reminder of how desperation can cloud judgment—and how only trial, error, patience and time can produce true epidemic control." Also see Conis, "Polio, DDT, and Disease Risk in the United States after World War II," https://www.journals.uchicago.edu/doi/abs/10.1093/envhis/emx086?journalCode=eh.

15 As cited in Engelbrecht et al., *Virus Mania*, 80.

16 West, *DDT Polio*, 17–22.

17 West, "Pesticides and Polio: A Critique of Scientific Literature," https://www.westonaprice.org/health-topics/environmental-toxins/pesticides-and-polio-a-critique-of-scientific-literature/#gsc.tab=0. Also see West, "Pesticides and Polio: A Critique of Scientific Literature," https://harvoa.org/polio/overview.htm#_edn4.

18 As noted by Engelbrecht et al., *Virus Mania*, 82.

19 Mayo Clinic, "Polio," https://www.mayoclinic.org/diseases-conditions/history-disease-outbreaks-vaccine-timeline/polio.

20 Humphries and Bystrianyk, *Dissolving Illusions*, 288.

21 As cited in Engdahl, "Toxicology vs Virology: Rockefeller Institute and the Criminal Polio Fraud," http://williamengdahl.com/englishNEO-12July2022.php.

22 West, *DDT Polio*, 15.

23 Lester and Parker, *What Really Makes You Ill*, 55.

24 Raj, "Polio free does not mean paralysis free," https://www.thehindu.com/opinion/lead/polio-free-does-not-mean-paralysis-free/article4266043.ece.

25 Lester and Parker, *What Really Makes You Ill*, 55.

26 Gear, "Nonpolio causes of polio-like paralytic syndromes," https://pubmed.ncbi.nlm.nih.gov/6740077/.

27 Tulp, "Experts say toxic pesticide DDT not linked to polio," https://apnews.com/article/fact-check-polio-vaccine-ddt-pesticide-480376540979.

28 Humphries and Bystrianyk, *Dissolving Illusions*, 288.

29 Maready, *The Moth in the Iron Lung*, 264–65.

30 Ibid., 265–66.

31 Ibid., 267.

32 Ibid., 263.

33 Huang, "THE SARS EPIDEMIC AND ITS AFTERMATH IN CHINA: A POLITICAL PERSPECTIVE," https://www.ncbi.nlm.nih.gov/books/NBK92479/.

34 World Health Organization, "Severe Acute Respiratory Syndrome (SARS)," https://www.who.int/health-topics/severe-acute-respiratory-syndrome#tab=tab_1.
35 Dr. Sam Bailey, "What Happened To SARS-1?" https://odysee.com/@drsambailey:c/what-happened-to-sars-1:8.
36 Engelbrecht et al., *Virus Mania*, 211.
37 Dr. Sam Bailey, "What Happened To SARS-1?" https://odysee.com/@drsambailey:c/what-happened-to-sars-1:8.
38 See Christine Massey's website: https://www.fluoridefreepeel.ca/fois-reveal-that-health-science-institutions-have-no-record-of-any-virus-having-been-isolated-purified-virology-isnt-a-science/. The CDC's response, in particular, can be found at the following link: https://www.fluoridefreepeel.ca/wp-content/uploads/2020/12/CDC-isolation-FOI-reply-any-coronavirus.pdf.
39 Kiuken et al., "Newly discovered coronavirus as the primary cause of severe acute respiratory syndrome," https://www.thelancet.com/journals/lancet/article/PIIS0140-6736(03)13967-0/fulltext.
40 Dr. Sam Bailey, "What Happened To SARS-1?" https://odysee.com/@drsambailey:c/what-happened-to-sars-1:8.
41 Fouchier, "Koch's postulates fulfilled for SARS virus," https://www.nature.com/articles/423240a/.
42 Dr. Tom Cowan, "HOW TO MAKE A POLIO VACCINE + A REBUTTAL – WEBINAR FROM AUGUST 30TH, 2023," https://www.bitchute.com/video/WaPyKutv4Oz9/. Dr. Cowan's request for properly controlled studies showing that "sick people make well people (or animals) sick" was the *first part* of a multipronged challenge. The other parts of the challenge are described in his video.
43 Ibid.
44 For a discussion on this topic, see Bailey, "A Farewell to Virology," 7.
45 Ibid.
46 As cited in Ibid., 40.
47 History, "Spanish Flu," https://www.history.com/topics/world-war-i/1918-flu-pandemic.
48 Rosenau, "Experiments to Determine Mode of Spread of Influenza," https://jamanetwork.com/journals/jama/article-abstract/221687. This conclusion is based off of the following statement in the paper: "The preliminary trials proved negative [so] we became bolder, and selecting nineteen of our volunteers, gave each one of them a very large quantity of a mixture of thirteen different strains of the Pfeiffer bacillus."
49 Ibid.
50 Ibid.
51 Ibid.
52 Ibid.
53 Ibid.
54 Ibid.
55 Ibid.

56 Ibid.
57 Ibid.
58 For example, see Rosenau, "Experiments upon volunteers to determine the cause and mode of spread of influenza, Boston, November and December, 1918," https://quod.lib.umich.edu/cgi/t/text/idx/f/flu/3750flu.0016.573/1/—experiments-upon-volunteers-to-determine-the-cause-and-mode?rgn=subject;view=image;q1=virology. Also see Engelbrecht et al., *Virus Mania*, 252.
59 Engelbrecht, et al., *Virus Mania*, 245–47.
60 Ibid., 247.
61 Ibid., 254.
62 McBean, *Swine Flu Expose*, chapter 2. See http://whale.to/vaccine/sf1.html. Also mentioned in Engelbrecht et al., 254–57.
63 As cited in Engelbrech et al., 258.
64 Firstenberg, *The Invisible Rainbow*, 91–92.
65 World Health Organization, "Current U.S. Bird Flu Situation in Humans," https://www.cdc.gov/flu/avianflu/inhumans.htm.
66 Engelbrecht, et al., *Virus Mania*, 214–15.
67 Ibid., 217–18.
68 Ibid., 231.
69 Ibid., 217–18.
70 Ibid., 231.
71 Killingley et al., "Use of a Human Influenza Challenge Model to Assess Person-to-Person Transmission: Proof-of Concept Study," https://academic.oup.com/jid/article/205/1/35/876311.
72 CDC, "What is Smallpox?" https://www.cdc.gov/smallpox/about/index.html.
73 Ibid.
74 Ibid.
75 See Christine Massey's website, https://www.fluoridefreepeel.ca/fois-reveal-that-health-science-institutions-have-no-record-of-any-virus-having-been-isolated-purified-virology-isnt-a-science/. The CDC's full FOIA response is available at https://www.fluoridefreepeel.ca/wp-content/uploads/2022/01/CDC-smallpox-PACKAGE-redacted.pdf.
76 *Find a Grave* website, "Dr Matthew Joseph Rodermund," https://www.findagrave.com/memorial/175430985/matthew-joseph-rodermund.
77 Hodge, *The Vaccine Superstition*, 57.
78 Ibid., 57–58.
79 Ibid., 59–60.
80 Ibid., 61.
81 *New York Times*, "Dr. Rodermund Escapes. Man Who Caused Smallpox Scare Gets Away from Appleton," https://timesmachine.nytimes.com/timesmachine/1901/01/28/102439229.html?pageNumber=8.
82 *The Vaccine Superstition*, Hodge, 63–64.
83 Koster, "SMALLPOX BLANKETS: MYTH OR MASSACRE?" https://www.historynet.com/smallpox-in-the-blankets/.

84 Lester and Parker, *What Really Makes You Ill*, 120.
85 Ibid., 121–22.
86 Ibid., 123.
87 From Hawden, "Truth," January 17, 1923, "Sanitation v. Vaccination: The Origin of Smallpox," https://www.soilandhealth.org/wp-content/uploads/GoodBooks/Hadwin-%20Table%20of%20Contents.pdf.
88 McBean, *The Poisoned Needle*, p. 1 of chapter 2.
89 Lester and Parker, *What Really Makes You Ill*, 49–50.
90 Humphries and Bystrianyk, *Dissolving Illusions*, 79.
91 Lester and Parker, *What Really Makes You Ill*, 51.
92 Ibid., 130.
93 Atti et al., "All that glitters is not gold: Mercury poisoning in a family mimicking an infectious illness," https://www.sciencedirect.com/science/article/abs/pii/S1538544220300183.
94 Czinn and Hoenig, "Poxes great and small: The stories behind their names," https://www.ncbi.nlm.nih.gov/pmc/articles/PMC9997050/.
95 Dr. Sam Bailey, "Chickenpox Parties and Varicella Zoster Virus?" https://drsambailey.com/resources/videos/viruses-unplugged/chickenpox-parties-and-varicella-zoster-virus/.
96 Hess, "Need of Further Research on the Transmissibility of Measles and Varicella," https://jamanetwork.com/journals/jama/article-abstract/222413?resultClick=1.
97 Dr. Sam Bailey, "Chickenpox Parties and Varicella Zoster Virus?" https://drsambailey.com/resources/videos/viruses-unplugged/chickenpox-parties-and-varicella-zoster-virus/.
98 Cowan and Morell, *The Truth about Contagion*, 77.
99 Dr. Sam Bailey, "What We Weren't Taught About Herpes," https://odysee.com/@drsambailey:c/What-We-Weren't-Taught-About-Herpes:3?src=embed.
100 Dr. Sam Bailey, "Chickenpox Parties and Varicella Zoster Virus?" https://drsambailey.com/resources/videos/viruses-unplugged/chickenpox-parties-and-varicella-zoster-virus/. She also makes reference to Dr. Thomas Cowen and Sally Fallon Morell's *The Contagion Myth (*renamed *The Truth about Contagion*), see p. 77 in the chapter on resonance.
101 Manek, "Do women's periods really sync up?" https://www.sciencefocus.com/the-human-body/do-periods-sync.
102 Helfrich-Förster et al., "Women temporarily synchronize their menstrual cycles with the luminance and gravimetric cycles of the Moon," https://pubmed.ncbi.nlm.nih.gov/33571128/.
103 For example, mentioned as a possibility by Dr. Marizelle Arce on a Twitter Space event on August 19, 2023: https://x.com/Censored4sure/status/1693077604150968379?s=20.
104 As discussed with Dr. Andrew Kaufman in personal correspondence on October 2, 2023.
105 Cowan and Morell, *The Truth about Contagion*, 77.

106 Dr. Sam Bailey, "Chickenpox Parties and Varicella Zoster Virus?" https://drsambailey.com/resources/videos/viruses-unplugged/chickenpox-parties-and-varicella-zoster-virus/.
107 CDC, "Cause and Transmission," https://www.cdc.gov/shingles/about/transmission.html.
108 Dr. Tom Cowan, "HOW TO MAKE A POLIO VACCINE + A REBUTTAL – WEBINAR FROM AUGUST 30TH, 2023," https://www.bitchute.com/video/WaPyKutv4Oz9/.
109 CDC, "What is Viral Hepatitis?" https://www.cdc.gov/hepatitis/abc/index.htm.
110 Dr. Sam Bailey, "What We Weren't Taught About Hepatitis," https://odysee.com/@drsambailey:c/What-We-Weren't-Taught-About-Hepatitis:4.
111 Ibid.
112 Ibid.
113 Ibid. Also see Engelbrecht et al., *Virus Mania*, chapter 4.
114 Ibid.
115 Kimble, "Pamela Anderson Announces She's Cured of Hepatitis C – See the Racy Photo She Posted to Celebrate," https://people.com/celebrity/pamela-anderson-is-cured-of-hep-c-see-the-photo-she-posted-to-celebrate/.
116 CDC, "Rabies in the U.S.," https://www.cdc.gov/rabies/location/usa/index.html.
117 Department of Health and Human Services, "FOIA Request to CDC re: purification of the 'rabies virus,'" https://www.fluoridefreepeel.ca/wp-content/uploads/2021/12/CDC-rabies-PACKAGE-redacted.pdf.
118 Geison, *The Private Science of Louis Pasteur*, 212–15. Also see Rappuoli, "1885, the first rabies vaccination in humans," https://www.pnas.org/doi/10.1073/pnas.1414226111.
119 Geison, *The Private Science of Louis Pasteur*, 227.
120 As cited in McBean, *The Poisoned Needle*, Addendum.
121 Geison, *The Private Science of Louis Pasteur*, 231.
122 Ibid.
123 As cited in McBean, *The Poisoned Needle*, Addendum. The text in *The Poisoned Needle* shows "3.000" rather than "3,000." This apparent typographical error in the primary source has been corrected here in the main text. Also, Morden's quote specifically refers to "hydrophobia." Morden further stated: "Is rabies then a disease? Have we isolated a virus or germ? Is the Pasteur-treatment specific? Is rabies, in short, fact or fancy? I believe it is fancy, for I have handled so-called rabid animals and humans without benefit of [the] Pasteur treatment and in no case has there been a death or any symptoms of rabies. I submit that rabies is non-existent and that the Pasteur treatment for rabies is worse than the disease, if it were a disease, which it is not."

124 CDC, "Vital Signs: Trends in Human Rabies Deaths and Exposures — United States, 1938–2018," https://www.cdc.gov/mmwr/volumes/68/wr/mm6823e1.htm.
125 As discussed in Dr. Sam Bailey, "What about Rabies?" https://odysee.com/@drsambailey:c/What-About-Rabies:a; referencing https://viroliegy.com/.
126 Viroliegy, "Exposing the lies of Germ Theory and virology using their own sources," https://viroliegy.com/2022/08/03/blindsided-by-rabies-with-michael-wallach-on-the-skeptico-podcast/.
127 Lester and Parker, *What Really Makes You Ill*, 170–71.
128 Dr. Sam Bailey, "What about Rabies?" https://odysee.com/@drsambailey:c/What-About-Rabies:a.
129 Grafe, *A History of Experimental Virology*, 5.
130 Ibid., 1.
131 World Health Organization, "Plague," https://www.who.int/news-room/fact-sheets/detail/plague.
132 Lester and Parker, *What Really Makes You Ill*, 143.
133 As cited in Ibid., 145.
134 As cited in Ibid., 146.
135 Engelbrecht et al., *Virus Mania*, 65–66.
136 Dr. Tom Cowan, "HOW TO MAKE A POLIO VACCINE + A REBUTTAL- WEBINAR FROM AUGUST 30TH, 2023," https://www.bitchute.com/video/WaPyKutv4Oz9/.

CHAPTER 5: VACCINE SAFETY

1 World Health Organization, "Immunization Agenda 2030: A Global Strategy to Leave No One Behind," https://www.who.int/teams/immunization-vaccines-and-biologicals/strategies/ia2030.
2 Charts are also available online at https://dissolvingillusions.com/graphs-images/#Charts. Also see the authors' detailed response to critiques at https://dissolvingillusions.com/critiques/.
3 Anonymous, *Turtles All the Way Down*, 269–70.
4 Rasmussen Reports, "COVID-19: Democratic Voters Support Harsh Measures Against Unvaccinated," https://www.rasmussenreports.com/public_content/politics/partner_surveys/jan_2022/covid_19_democratic_voters_support_harsh_measures_against_unvaccinated.
5 Goel, "Facebook widens ban on vaccine misinformation," https://www.cbsnews.com/news/facebook-widens-ban-on-vaccine-misinformation-to-include-anti-vaccination-conspiracy-theories/.
6 Pruitt-Young, "YouTube Is Banning All Content That Spreads Vaccine Misinformation," https://www.npr.org/2021/09/29/1041493544/youtube-vaccine-misinformation-ban.
7 Zakrzewski and Menn, "5th Circuit finds Biden White House, CDC likely violated First Amendment," https://www.washingtonpost.com/technology/2023/09/08/5th-circuit-ruling-covid-content-moderation/.

8 War Room/DailyClout, "Pfizer Document Analysis Reports," summary chapter.
9 Ibid.
10 Anonymous, *Turtles All the Way Down*, 514.
11 INSTITUTE FOR AUTISM SCIENCE AND THE INFORMED CONSENT ACTION NETWORK vs. CENTERS FOR DISEASE CONTROL AND PREVENTION, 6, https://www.icandecide.org/wp-content/uploads/2020/03/001-COMPLAINT-against-Centers-for-Disease-Control-and-Prevention.pdf.
12 Cornell Law School, 42 U.S. Code § 300aa–11 – Petitions for compensation, https://www.law.cornell.edu/uscode/text/42/300aa-11. Also discussed on page 1 of the lawsuit referenced above, available at https://icandecide.org/wp-content/uploads/2020/03/001-COMPLAINT-against-Centers-for-Disease-Control-and-Prevention.pdf.
13 Kennedy Jr. and Hooker, *Vax-Unvax*, 1.
14 INSTITUTE FOR AUTISM SCIENCE AND THE INFORMED CONSENT ACTION NETWORK vs. CENTERS FOR DISEASE CONTROL AND PREVENTION, 9, https://www.icandecide.org/wp-content/uploads/2020/03/001-COMPLAINT-against-Centers-for-Disease-Control-and-Prevention.pdf.
15 Ibid.
16 HRSA, "Data and Statistics," https://www.hrsa.gov/sites/default/files/hrsa/vicp/vicp-stats-09-01-23.pdf.
17 Harvard Pilgrim Health Care, Inc., Electronic Support for Public Health–Vaccine Adverse Event Reporting System (ESP:VAERS), https://digital.ahrq.gov/sites/default/files/docs/publication/r18hs017045-lazarus-final-report-2011.pdf.
18 Ibid.
19 CDC, "Vaccine Excipient Summary," https://www.cdc.gov/vaccines/pubs/pinkbook/downloads/appendices/B/excipient-table-2.pdf?mibextid=Zxz2cZ.
20 Children's Hospital of Philadelphia, "Vaccine Ingredients – Fetal Tissues," https://www.chop.edu/centers-programs/vaccine-education-center/vaccine-ingredients/fetal-tissues# and https://www.youtube.com/watch?v=PhIvTBZzfsI&list=PLUv9oht3hC6TTY-k6FbWQDWS-aR-KGRGZ&index=15.
21 ATSDR, "Formaldehyde and Your Health," https://www.atsdr.cdc.gov/formaldehyde/.
22 National Institute of Environmental Health Sciences, "Formaldehyde," https://www.niehs.nih.gov/health/topics/agents/formaldehyde/index.cfm.
23 Centers for Disease Control and Prevention, "What's in Vaccines?" https://www.cdc.gov/vaccines/vac-gen/additives.htm.
24 Also see Olmstead and Blaxill, *The Age of Autism: Mercury, Medicine, and a Man-Made Epidemic*.

25 CDC, "Thimerosal and Vaccines," https://www.cdc.gov/vaccinesafety/concerns/thimerosal/index.html.
26 Dr. Sam Bailey, "Aluminium, Vaccines & Detox," https://odysee.com/@drsambailey:c/Aluminium-Vaccines-Detox:a?src=embed.
27 CDC, "Adjuvants and Vaccines," https://www.cdc.gov/vaccinesafety/concerns/adjuvants.html.
28 Informed Consent Action Network, "NIH Concedes It Has No Studies Assessing The Safety Of Injecting Aluminum," https://icandecide.org/article/nih-concedes-it-has-no-studies-assessing-the-safety-of-injecting-aluminum-adjuvants/.
29 Department of Health and Human Services, "Re: FOIA Case Number: 50822, and HHS Appeal No.: 19-0083-AA," https://www.icandecide.org/wp-content/uploads/2020/08/20190719-HHS-Final-Response-IR0084-Appeal.pdf.
30 Niu, "Overview of the Relationship Between Aluminum Exposure and Health of Human Being," https://pubmed.ncbi.nlm.nih.gov/30315446/.
31 Exley, "The toxicity of aluminum in humans," https://www.sciencedirect.com/science/article/abs/pii/S1286011516000023. Also cited in Dr. Sam Bailey, "Aluminium, Vaccines & Detox," https://odysee.com/@drsambailey:c/Aluminium-Vaccines-Detox:a?src=embed.
32 Anonymous, *Turtles All the Way Down*, 81.
33 Siri, "Proof Regarding the Clinical Trials Relied Upon by the FDA to License the Childhood Vaccines on the CDC Childhood Vaccine Schedule," https://aaronsiri.substack.com/p/what-the-casual-cruelty-of-dr-paul.
34 Anonymous, *Turtles All the Way Down*, 57.
35 Siri, "Proof Regarding the Clinical Trials Relied Upon by the FDA to License the Childhood Vaccines on the CDC Childhood Vaccine Schedule," https://aaronsiri.substack.com/p/what-the-casual-cruelty-of-dr-paul.
36 Anonymous, *Turtles All the Way Down*, 76.
37 Kennedy Jr. and Hooker, *Vax-Unvax*, 8. Dr. Andrew Kaufman also noted in personal correspondence with the author on October 2, 2023, that drugs like antibiotics and psychiatric drugs do use true placebo-controlled trials. However, as noted on cancer.net, cancer drugs are more problematic: "It is important to know that whenever a placebo is used in a cancer clinical trial, people who receive the placebo will also receive the standard treatment for the specific cancer as well." See https://www.cancer.net/research-and-advocacy/clinical-trials/placebos-cancer-clinical-trials.
38 Kennedy Jr. and Hooker, *Vax-Unvax*, 3.
39 Ibid.
40 Bigtree, in the foreword to Kennedy Jr. and Hooker, *Vax-Unvax*, xvi–ii.
41 As cited in Ibid., xvii.
42 As cited in Kennedy Jr. and Hooker, *Vax-Unvax*, 4.

43 Ibid.
44 Package insert, "ENERGIX-B," https://www.fda.gov/media/119403/download.
45 From the author's personal correspondence with Dr. Andrew Kaufman on October 3, 2023.
46 Kennedy Jr. and Hooker, *Vax-Unvax*, xvii.
47 Ibid, 37.
48 Ibid., 5.

CHAPTER 6: PHYSICALISM VS. IDEALISM

1 For more on these arguments, see the work of Dr. Bernardo Kastrup—for instance, *The Idea of the World.* Also discussed in my books *An End to Upside Down Thinking* and *An End to Upside Down Living.*
2 Kastrup, *The Idea of the World*, 21.
3 Ibid., 131. Also see Kelly, "Best way forward or unnecessary detour? A review of 'Dual-Aspect Monism and the Deep Structure of Meaning,'" https://www.essentiafoundation.org/best-way-forward-or-unnecessary-detour-a-review-of-dual-aspect-monism-and-the-deep-structure-of-meaning/reading/.
4 Described in Kastrup, *Why Materialism Is Baloney*, for example.
5 Kastrup et al., "Disorder Explain Life, the Universe and Everything?" https://blogs.scientificamerican.com/observations/could-multiple-personality-disorder-explain-life-the-universe-and-everything/.
6 Interview with Max Planck, *The Observer* (1931).
7 Schrödinger, *What Is Life? with Mind and Matter*, 139.
8 Radin, *Real Magic*, 197, 205.
9 This notion is often discussed by Rupert Spira, a spiritual philosopher.
10 For more elaborate explanation of the "hard problem," see The Internet Encyclopedia of Mind, "The Hard Problem of Consciousness," https://iep.utm.edu/hard-problem-of-conciousness/.
11 I first heard this analogy—with regard to consciousness and the brain—described by Dr. Bernardo Kastrup. For example, see *Where Is My Mind?* podcast.
12 This analogy has been described by many consciousness researchers, such as Dr. Larry Dossey. See *An End to Upside Down Thinking* for more on this subject.
13 As referenced in my previous books and my podcast series *Where Is My Mind?*, available at https://podcasts.apple.com/us/podcast/where-is-my-mind/id1470129415.
14 For example, see, Rawlette, "Does an Afterlife Obviously Exist?" https://www.psychologytoday.com/gb/blog/mysteries-consciousness/202204/does-afterlife-obviously-exist.
15 See my book *An End to Upside Down Thinking* for more information on near-death experiences.
16 Ibid.

17 For example, see Kastrup and Kelly, "Misreporting and Confirmation Bias in Psychedelic Research," https://blogs.scientificamerican.com/observations/misreporting-and-confirmation-bias-in-psychedelic-research/.
18 See Gober, *An End to Upside Down Thinking*, chapter 2. Also see the *Where Is My Mind?* podcast.
19 Kastrup, *The Idea of the World*, 175.
20 Kastrup, "Transcending the Brain," https://blogs.scientificamerican.com/guest-blog/transcending-the-brain/.
21 See Dr. Radin's website for more information on a wide variety of studies: https://www.deanradin.com/publications.
22 Williams, "Revisiting the ganzfeld ESP debate: A basic review and assessment," https://www.researchgate.net/publication/280019566_Revisiting_the_Ganzfeld_ESP_Debate_A_Basic_Review_and_Assessment.
23 See Dean Radin's books *Supernormal, Entangled Minds*, and *The Conscious Universe*. Also see Tressoldi, "Extraordinary claims require extraordinary evidence: The case of non-local perception, a classical and Bayesian review of evidences."
24 Mossbridge, Tressoldi & Utts, "Predictive physiological anticipation preceding seemingly unpredictable stimuli: A meta-analysis"; Bem, Tressoldi, Raberyon, & Duggan, "Feeling the future: A meta-analysis of 90 experiments on the anomalous anticipation of random future events."
25 Bosch, Steinkamp & Boller, "Examining psychokinesis: The interaction of human intention with random number generators—a meta-analysis; Radin, Nelson, Dobyns, & Houtkooper, "Re-examining psychokinesis: Commentary on the Bösch, Steinkamp and Boller metaanalysis"; Nelson, Radin, Shoup, and Bancel, "Correlations of continuous random data with major world events"; global-mind.org/results.html.
26 Radin, *Real Magic*, 97.
27 The following study references a 30 percent vs. 25 percent differential among the studies examined: Williams, "Revisiting the ganzfeld ESP debate: A basic review and assessment," https://www.researchgate.net/publication/280019566_Revisiting_the_Ganzfeld_ESP_Debate_A_Basic_Review_and_Assessment. In *Where Is My Mind?* podcast, Ep. 3: Telepathy, the scientists interviewed discussed slightly higher hit rates (32 or 33 percent). The exact figures vary depending on the bundle of studies chosen, but the general trend emerges clearly: something is going on that traditional science cannot explain.
28 See chapter 4 of Gober, *An End to Upside Down Thinking*. Also see Ep. 4: CIA Psychic Spying and Knowing the Future of the *Where Is My Mind?* podcast for more information on remote viewing.
29 Cardeña, Etzel. "The experimental evidence for parapsychological phenomena: A review," https://doi.org/10.1037/amp0000236.

30 Utts, "An Assessment of the Evidence for Psychic Functioning," https://www.ics.uci.edu/~jutts/air.pdf. Also available in the *Journal of Parapsychology*.
31 For instance, see *The Self Does Not Die* (second edition) by Rivas et al.
32 See *Where Is My Mind?* podcast, Ep. 2: Blindfolded.
33 Greyson, "Seeing Dead People Not Known to Have Died: "Peak in Darien" Experiences," https://anthrosource.onlinelibrary.wiley.com/doi/abs/10.1111/j.1548-1409.2010.01064.x.
34 Greyson and van Lommel, "Critique of Recent Report of Electrical Activity in the Dying Human Brain," https://iands.org/images/stories/pdf_downloads/vanLommel-Greyson-2023-Critique-Recent-Report-Electrical-Activity-Dying-Human-Brain.pdf. Also see Greyson, van Lommel, and Fenwick, "Recent Report of Electroencephalogram of a Dying Human Brain," https://www.iands.org/images/stories/pdf_downloads/Greyson_et_al-2022-Commentary-on-Report-of-EEG-in-a-Dying-Human-Brain.pdf.
35 Greyson, *After*, 110.
36 Ibid., 111.
37 Shared Crossing Research Initiative, "Shared Death Experiences: A Little-Known Type of End-of-Life Phenomena Reported by Caregivers and Loved Ones," https://pubmed.ncbi.nlm.nih.gov/33813876/.
38 See Gober, *An End to Upside Down Thinking*, chapters 10 and 11. Also see the peer-reviewed research from the Windbridge Research Center, https://www.windbridge.org/research/.
39 See Division of Perceptual Studies, "Children Who Remember Previous Lives – Academic Publications," https://med.virginia.edu/perceptual-studies/publications/academic-publications/children-who-remember-previous-lives-academic-publications/.

CHAPTER 7: CONSCIOUSNESS, HEALTH, AND DISEASE

1 "The End of COVID" also discusses many fascinating possibilities that should be studied further. See https://theendofcovid.com/.
2 Bosch, Steinkamp & Boller, "Examining psychokinesis: The interaction of human intention with random number generators—a meta-analysis"; Radin, Nelson, Dobyns & Houtkooper, "Re-examining psychokinesis: Commentary on the Bösch, Steinkamp and Boller metaanalysis"; Nelson, Radin, Shoup, and Bancel, "Correlations of continuous random data with major world events"; global-mind.org/results.html.
3 Princeton Engineering Anomalies Research, http://pearlab.icrl.org/.
4 The Global Consciousness Project, http://www.global-mind.org/.
5 Jain, *Healing Ourselves*, 68–77.
6 Raypole, "What Is the Nocebo Effect?" https://www.healthline.com/health/nocebo-effect#how-it-works.
7 Radin, *Supernormal*, 110–14.

8 Bengston et al., "Differential In Vivo Effects on Cancer Models by Recorded Magnetic Signals Derived From a Healing Technique," https://pubmed.ncbi.nlm.nih.gov/37325440/.
9 Ibid.
10 Haberer, *Healer: The Jerry Wills Story*, back cover.
11 Ibid., xxii.
12 jerrywills, "Jerry Wills on FOX 2006," https://www.youtube.com/watch?v=J0e7uUPtALs.
13 Gladstone, *Miracle Soul Healer*, 3.
14 Ibid., 293.
15 Ibid., 40.
16 Ibid., 42.
17 Ibid., 107–08.
18 Ibid., 89–90.
19 Jain, *Healing Ourselves*, 18–19.
20 Ibid., 115–130. "Mock" healings were also part of Dr. Jain's methodology.
21 Ibid., 124.
22 Ibid., 117.
23 Ibid., 119–20.
24 Ibid., 131–32.
25 McKusick, *Electric Body, Electric Health*, 20.
26 Jain, *Healing Ourselves*, 90–91.
27 Ibid., 95–96.
28 Ibid., 102–03.
29 See Gober, *An End to Upside Down Thinking*, chapter 3.
30 HeartMath Institute, *Science of the Heart*, 42.
31 Ibid.
32 Ibid.
33 See the *Where Is My Mind?* podcast interview with Dr. Larry Dossey, which is also featured in Ep. 3: Telepathy. For more on telesomatic events, see *An End to Upside Down Thinking*, 86–87.
34 Ibid.
35 Rozman, in *Heart Intelligence*, 226–27.
36 Backster, *Primary Perception*, 11.
37 Ibid., 24.
38 Ibid., 23.
39 Ibid., 29.
40 Ibid., 98.
41 Ibid., 99.
42 Ibid., 101.
43 Ibid., 112.
44 Ibid., 113.
45 Ibid., 115.
46 Pearsall, *The Heart's Code*, 7.
47 Ibid., 90.

48 Ibid., 89.
49 Ibid., 83.
50 IONS, "Spontaneous Remission: An Annotated Bibliography," https://noetic.org/publication/spontaneous-remission-annotated-bibliography/.
51 Anita Moorjani, "THE DAY MY LIFE CHANGED: February 2, 2006," https://www.anitamoorjani.com/my-nde.
52 Moorjani, *Dying to Be Me*, 71–72 (Kindle).
53 Ibid.
54 Ibid., 73 (Kindle).
55 Ibid., 75–76 (Kindle).
56 Ibid., 89 (Kindle).
57 Sunfellow, "Near-Death Experiences & Miraculous Healings," https://sunfellow.substack.com/p/near-death-experiences-and-miraculous.
58 Hawkins, *Letting Go*, 299.
59 Ibid., 305.
60 Ibid., 311.
61 Hawkins, *Healing and Recovery*, 64–65.
62 Willow, *German New Medicine*, 15.
63 Markolin, "THE FIVE BIOLOGICAL LAWS OF THE NEW MEDICINE," https://learninggnm.com/SBS/documents/five_laws.html.
64 Ibid.
65 Reclamation Radio with Kelly Brogan MD, "Why German New Medicine with Dr. Melissa Sell," https://podcasts.apple.com/us/podcast/reclamation-radio-with-kelly-brogan-md/id1663947298?i=1000622254539.
66 Stevenson, *Children Who Remember Previous Lives*, 12.
67 Stevenson, *Where Reincarnation and Biology Intersect*, 2.
68 Ibid., 7.
69 Ibid.
70 Healing Powers, "Mira Kelley and Past Lives," https://music.amazon.co.uk/podcasts/5698afd2-031d-400b-853f-b51d96770612/episodes/3496420b-cbf3-496a-9cb4-53bd278bbd59/healing-powers-podcast-mira-kelley-and-past-lives.
71 Sharma and Tucker, "Cases of the Reincarnation Type with Memories from the Intermission Between Lives," 1. https://med.virginia.edu/perceptual-studies/wp-content/uploads/sites/360/2015/11/Intermission-memories-JNDS.pdf.
72 Schwartz, *Your Soul's Plan*, 31.
73 For more information on ritual abuse, see Gober, *An End to Upside Down Contact*, chapter 2.
74 Faith-Masterson, *I Am Serena*, 19.
75 Rupert Sheldrake, "Morphic Resonance: Research and Papers," https://www.sheldrake.org/research/morphic-resonance.

76 For an overview of family constellation therapy, see GoodTherapy, "Family Constellations," https://www.goodtherapy.org/learn-about-therapy/types/family-constellations.
77 Wahbeh, "A mixed methods phenomenological and exploratory study of channeling."
78 Gallagher, *Demonic Foes*, 7.
79 Ibid., 11.
80 Ibid., 9.
81 Ibid., 25.
82 Ibid., 11.
83 TLM4Columbia, "Voices in Virtue Lectures: Fr. Chad Ripperger — Demonology Function & Psychology," https://www.youtube.com/watch?v=A4Aq7WGIhzA.
84 Grafe, *A History of Experimental Virology*, 3–5.
85 See I Am Serena, "FREE BREATHING," https://www.iamserena.net/breath/. Breathing exercise 11 discusses Norma Delaney's Kwan Yin breathing method (alternatively spelled Quan Yen).
86 See Gober, *An End to Upside Down Contact*, chapter 7.
87 For more on this topic see Gober, *An End to Upside Down Contact*. Also see the *Eden* series by Paul Wallis.

CONCLUSION: WHAT'S AT STAKE

1 The term *medical-industrial complex* is often invoked in contemporary discussions about medicine, but one historical example of its use is from a 1980 article in *The New England Journal of Medicine* by Arnold Relman, MD, titled "The New Medical-Industrial Complex." The abstract states: "The most important health-care development of the day is the recent, relatively unheralded rise of a huge new industry that supplies health-care services for profit. Proprietary hospitals and nursing homes, diagnostic laboratories, home-care and emergency-room services, hemodialysis, and a wide variety of other services produced a gross income to this industry last year of about $35 billion to $40 billion. This new 'medical-industrial complex' may be more efficient than its nonprofit competition, but it creates the problems of overuse and fragmentation of services, overemphasis on technology, and 'cream-skimming,' and it may also exercise undue influence on national health policy."
2 As mentioned by Dr. Thomas Cowan, "The Infectious Myth - Thomas Cowan on COVID-19 and Germ Theory," https://podcasts.apple.com/us/podcast/the-infectious-myth/id829019119?i=1000476566837.
3 Williams, *Terrain Therapy*, 25.
4 Jain, *Healing Ourselves*, 57.
5 Dr. Thomas Cowan has often referenced this method of getting to the truth: figuring out what's not true, thereby leaving a smaller possibility set of what *is* true. In Indian spiritual traditions this approach is known as "neti neti" (not this, not that).

6 See Lester and Parker, *What Really Makes You Ill?*, 686–735.

7 For example, see *SuperWellness* by Dr. Edith Ubuntu Chan. Regarding water, many practitioners speak about the importance of "structured" water. See, for example, the work of Gerald Pollack, PhD, and his book titled *The Fourth Phase of Water: Beyond Solid Liquid Vapor*. Also, for more on blue light, see Harvard Health Publishing, "Blue light has a dark side," https://www.health.harvard.edu/staying-healthy/blue-light-has-a-dark-side.

8 See Gober, *An End to the Upside Down Reset*, chapter 7.

9 A review by Bobby Matherne, "The Fall of the Spirits of Darkness, GA#177 14 Lectures in Dornach in 1917 by Rudolf Steiner," http://www.doyletics.com/arj/falldark.pdf. Also in Steiner, *The Fall of the Spirits of Darkness*, 85, 199–200.

10 Plescia, "Are We Prepared for the Next Pandemic? Anthony Fauci Weighs In at AHIP," https://medcitynews.com/2023/06/fauci-covid-pandemic-vaccines-public-health/.

11 For example, see BBC News, "Howard Springs: Australia police arrest quarantine escapees," https://www.bbc.com/news/world-australia-59486285; Jordan, "In Texas, a Quarantine Camp for Migrants With Covid-19," https://www.nytimes.com/2021/08/12/us/coronavirus-migrants-border-covid.html; and Brady, "Three military camps will be adapted into isolation units to help deal with Covid surge," https://www.independent.ie/irish-news/three-military-camps-will-be-adapted-into-isolation-units-to-help-deal-with-covid-surge/39941068.html.

12 JeffMara Podcast, "Man Struck By Lighting; DIED & Was Told The Future (NDE) | Dannion Brinkley," https://youtu.be/l1HasR5er3c.

13 Thomas Friese, in the preface to Jünger, *The Forest Passage*. The quotation was mentioned by Dr. Tom Cowan, "A LOOK AT MALARIA – WEBINAR FROM JULY 12TH, 2023," https://www.bitchute.com/video/SvHsnKFkJH4O/?list=notifications&randomize=false.

BIBLIOGRAPHY

Abramson, John, and Barbara Starfield. "The Effect of Conflict of Interest on Biomedical Research and Clinical Practice Guidelines: Can We Trust the Evidence in Evidence-Based Medicine?" *J Am Board Fam Pract*. Sept.–Oct. 2005; 18(5): 414–18. https://www.jabfm.org/content/jabfp/18/5/414.full.pdf.

AetherMedia22 Tony Punch. "Dr. Suzanne Humphries Lecture on Vaccines & Health! MY ADVICE YOU DIDNT ASK FOR, PAY CLOSE ATTENTION TO THIS ONE!!!" Rumble video, January 2023. https://rumble.com/v24n1vi-dr.-suzanne-humphries-lecture-on-vaccine-and-health-my-advice-pay-close-att.html.

Ahmad et al. "Provisional Mortality Data—United States, 2022." CDC website, May 5, 2023. https://www.cdc.gov/mmwr/volumes/72/wr/mm7218a3.htm.

AIDSTruth. "HIV heterosexual transmission and the "Padian paper myth." AIDSTruth website, n.d. https://aidstruth.org/misuse-of-studies/padian/.

Al-Bayati et al. "To: Bruce Alberts, Editor in Chief, Science." December 1, 2018. https://garynull.com/wp-content/uploads/2023/08/081201-Letter-To-Science-Gallo-Papers.pdf.

Almeida, June, and D.A.J. Tyrrell. "The Morphology of Three Previously Uncharacterized Human Respiratory Viruses That

Grow in Organ Culture." *Journal of General Virology*, April 1, 1967. https://www.microbiologyresearch.org/content/journal/jgv/10.1099/0022-1317-1-2-175.

Anonymous. *Turtles All the Way Down: Vaccine Science and Myth.* The Turtles Team, 2022.

Ashfield, Rebecca et al. (Ed.). *Vaccinology and Methods in Vaccine Research.* London: Academic Press, 2022.

ATSDR. "Formaldehyde and Your Health." ATSDR website, February 10, 2016. https://www.atsdr.cdc.gov/formaldehyde/.

Atti, Sukhshant et al. "All that glitters is not gold: Mercury poisoning in a family mimicking an infectious illness." *Current Problems in Pediatric and Adolescent Health Care*, February 2020; 50(2). https://www.sciencedirect.com/science/article/abs/pii/S1538544220300183.

Backster, Cleve. *Primary Perception: Biocommunication with Plants, Living Foods, and Human Cells.* Anza: White Rose Millenium Press, 2003.

Bailey, Mark. "A Farewell to Virology," (Expert Edition). Dr. Sam Bailey website, September 15, 2022. https://drsambailey.com/a-farewell-to-virology-expert-edition/.

Bailey, Mark, and John Bevan-Smith. *The COVID-19 Fraud & War on Humanity.* Dr. Sam Bailey website, November 11, 2021. https://drsambailey.com/the-covid-19-fraud-war-on-humanity/.

Balthazar, Axel (E.D.). *Project MK-ULTRA and Mind Control Technology.* Kempton: Adventures Unlimited Press, 2017.

Banks, Nancy Turner. *AIDS, Opium, Diamonds, and Empire: The Deadly Virus of International Greed.* New York: iUniverse, 2010.

BBC News. "Howard Springs: Australia police arrest quarantine escapees." BBC News, December 1, 2021. https://www.bbc.com/news/world-australia-59486285.

Bech, V. "Studies on measles virus in monkey kidney tissue cultures." *Acta Pathol Microbiol Scand.* 1958;42(1): 86–96. https://pubmed.ncbi.nlm.nih.gov/13508251/.

Bech, V. and P. von Magnus. "Studies on measles virus in monkey kidney tissue cultures." *Acta Pathol Microbiol Scand.* 1958;42(1): 75–85. https://pubmed.ncbi.nlm.nih.gov/13508250/.

Bem, Daryl et al. "Feeling the Future: A Meta-Analysis of 90 Experiments on the Anomalous Anticipation of Random Future Events." *F1000 Research* 4 (2015): 1188. https://f1000research.com/articles/4-1188/v1.

BenGreenfield Life. "Ben's New Dietary Protocol, Vegetables Vs. Viruses, Whether Viruses Really Exist & Much More With Dr. Thomas Cowan." BenGreenfield Life website, August 3, 2023. https://bengreenfieldlife.com/podcast/tom-cowan-podcast/.

Bengston, William et al. "Differential In Vivo Effects on Cancer Models by Recorded Magnetic Signals Derived From a Healing Technique." *Dose Response*, June 2, 2023;21(2). https://pubmed.ncbi.nlm.nih.gov/37325440/.

Bosch, Holger, Fiona Steinkamp, and Emil Boller. "Examining Psychokinesis: The Interaction of Human Intention with Random Number Generators; A Meta-Analysis." *Psychological Bulletin* 132, no. 4 (2006): 497–523.

Bown, Stephen. *Scurvy: How a Surgeon, a Mariner and a Gentleman Solved the Greatest Medical Mystery of the Age of Sail.* New York: Thomas Dunne Books, 2003.

Britannica. "Antonie van Leeuwenhoek." Britannica website, August 22, 2023. https://www.britannica.com/biography/Antonie-van-Leeuwenhoek.

Britannica. "Beriberi." Britannica website, September 13, 2023. https://www.britannica.com/science/beriberi.

Britannica. "History of optical microscopes." Britannica website, n.d. https://www.britannica.com/technology/microscope/History-of-optical-microscopes.

Britannica. "Louis Pasteur." Britannica website. https://www.britannica.com/biography/Louis-Pasteur.

Britannica. "Pellagra." Britannica website, July 28, 2023. https://www.britannica.com/science/pellagra.

Britannica. "Endotoxin." Britannica website, n.d. https://www.britannica.com/science/endotoxin.

Britannica ProCon.org. "FDA-Approved Prescription Drugs Later Pulled from the Market by the FDA." Britannica ProCon.org website, December 1, 2021. https://prescriptiondrugs.procon.org/fda-approved-prescription-drugs-later-pulled-from-the-market/.

Britannica. "Vaccine development of Louis Pasteur." Britannica website, n.d. https://www.britannica.com/biography/Louis-Pasteur/Vaccine-development.

Broad Institute. "David Baltimore, Ph.D." Broad Institute website, n.d. https://www.broadinstitute.org/bios/david-baltimore.

Brownstein, Barry. "Google Is Burying Alternative Health Sites to Protect People from 'Dangerous' Medical Advice." *FEE Stories*, August 6, 2019. https://fee.org/articles/google-is-burying-alternative-health-sites-to-protect-people-from-dangerous-medical-advice/.

Bryson, Christopher. *The Fluoride Deception*. New York: Seven Stories Press, 2004.

Bullock et al. "Difficulties in Differentiating Coronaviruses from Subcellular Structures in Human Tissues by Electron Microscopy." CDC website, April 2021. https://wwwnc.cdc.gov/eid/article/27/4/20-4337_article.

Burdick, Suzanne. "4 Studies Add to Evidence of Wireless Technology-Related Electromagnetic Radiation in Humans." Children's Health Defense website, January 18, 2023. https://childrenshealthdefense.org/defender/wireless-technology-electromagnetic-radiation-humans/.

Caley, Leon et al. "The FDA-approved drug ivermectin inhibits the replication of SARS-CoV-2 in vitro." *Antiviral Research*, 178 (2020). https://doi.org/10.1016/j.antiviral.2020.104787

Cancer.net. "Placebos in Cancer Clinical Trials." Cancer.net website, October 2022. https://www.cancer.net/research-and-advocacy/clinical-trials/placebos-cancer-clinical-trials.

Cardeña, Etzel. "The experimental evidence for parapsychological phenomena: A review." *American Psychologist*, 73(5) (2018), 663–77. https://doi.org/10.1037/amp0000236.

Carson, Rachel. *Silent Spring*. New York: Mariner Books, 1962.

Carter, John, and Venetia Saunders. *Virology: Principles and Applications*. West Sussex: Wiley, 2013.

Cassol, Clarissa et al. "Appearances Can Be Deceiving—Viral-like Inclusions in COVID-19 Negative Renal Biopsies by Electron Microscopy." *Kidney360* 1: 824–28, 2020.

CDC, "Adjuvants and Vaccines," CDC website, September 27, 2022. https://www.cdc.gov/vaccinesafety/concerns/adjuvants.html.

CDC. "Cause and Transmission." CDC website, n.d. https://www.cdc.gov/shingles/about/transmission.html.

CDC. "Chronic Diseases in America." CDC website, n.d. https://www.cdc.gov/chronicdisease/resources/infographic/chronic-diseases.htm.

CDC. "History of Smallpox." CDC website, n.d. https://www.cdc.gov/smallpox/history/history.html.

CDC. "Rabies in the U.S." CDC website, n.d. https://www.cdc.gov/rabies/location/usa/index.html.

CDC. "Thimerosal and Vaccines." CDC website, August 25, 2020. https://www.cdc.gov/vaccinesafety/concerns/thimerosal/index.html.

CDC. "Vaccine Excipient Summary." November 1, 2021. https://www.cdc.gov/vaccines/pubs/pinkbook/downloads/appendices/B/excipient-table-2.pdf?mibextid=Zxz2cZ.

CDC. "Vital Signs: Trends in Human Rabies Deaths and Exposures—United States, 1938–2018." CDC website, June 14, 2019; 68(23), 524–28. https://www.cdc.gov/mmwr/volumes/68/wr/mm6823e1.htm.

CDC. "What is Polio?" CDC website, January 9, 2023. https://www.cdc.gov/polio/what-is-polio/index.htm.

CDC. "What is Smallpox?" CDC website, June 7, 2016. https://www.cdc.gov/smallpox/about/index.html.

CDC. "What is Viral Hepatitis?" CDC website, n.d. https://www.cdc.gov/hepatitis/abc/index.htm.

CDC, "What's in Vaccines?" CDC website, July 14, 2022. https://www.cdc.gov/vaccines/vac-gen/additives.htm.

Chan, Edith Ubuntu. *SuperWellness: Become Your Own Best Healer*. San Francisco: School of Dan Tian Wellness, 2017.

Childre et al. *Heart Intelligence: Connecting with the Heart's Intuitive Guidance for Effective Choices and Solutions*. Cardiff-by-the-Sea, CA: Waterside Productions, 2022.

Children's Hospital of Philadelphia. "Vaccine Ingredients – Fetal Tissues." n.d. https://www.chop.edu/centers-programs/vaccine-education-center/vaccine-ingredients/fetal-tissues# and https://www.youtube.com/watch?v=PhIvTBZzfsI&list=PLUv9oht3hC6TTY-k6FbWQDWS-aR-KGRGZ&index=15.

ChrisMasseyFOIs. "OFFICIAL EVIDENCE THAT VIROLOGY IS PSEUDOSCIENCE – CHRISTINE MASSEY JUNE 10 2023." Bitchute video, June 10, 2023. https://www.bitchute.com/video/gvu4NbieSuVb/.

Cleveland Clinic. "Staph Infection." Cleveland Clinic website, n.d. https://my.clevelandclinic.org/health/diseases/21165-staph-infection-staphylococcus-infection.

Conis, Elena. "A misfire in fighting polio provides clues as to how we'll beat covid." *Washington Post*, April 14, 2022. https://www.washingtonpost.com/outlook/2022/04/14/misfire-fighting-polio-provides-clues-how-well-beat-covid/

Conis, Elena. "Polio, DDT, and Disease Risk in the United States after World War II." *The Environmental History*, 2017; 22(4). https://www.journals.uchicago.edu/doi/abs/10.1093/envhis/emx086?journalCode=eh.

Connett, Paul et al. *The Cause Against Fluoride: How Hazardous Waste Ended Up in Our Drinking Water and the Bad Science and Powerful Politics That Keep It There*. White River Junction, VT: Chelsea Green Publishing, 2010.

Corrochio, Eduardo. "Kary Mullis Explains the PCR Test." YouTube video, October 4, 2020. https://www.youtube.com/watch?v=ZmZft4fXhQQ.

Cowan, Thomas. *Breaking the Spell: The Scientific Evidence for Ending the COVID Delusion*. Thomas S. Cowan, MD, 2021.

Cowan, Thomas, and Sally Fallon Morell. *The Truth about Contagion: Exploring Theories of How Disease Spreads*. New York: Skyhorse Publishing, 2021.

Creative Artists Uniting for the Sovereignty of Everyone. "Alec Zeck | C.A.U.S.E Fest Nashville 2023." Rumble video, August

2023. https://rumble.com/v35zsqe-alec-zeck-c.a.u.s.e-fest-nashville-2023.html.

Crosta, Peter. "Everything you need to know about scurvy." *Medical-NewsToday*, February 16, 2023. https://www.medicalnewstoday.com/articles/155758.

Culshaw, Rebecca. *The Real AIDS Epidemic: How the Tragic HIV Mistake Threatens Us All.* New York: Skyhorse Publishing, 2023.

Czinn, Amber, and Leonard Hoenig. "Poxes great and small: The stories behind their names." *Clin Dermatol*, March 9, 2023. https://www.ncbi.nlm.nih.gov/pmc/articles/PMC9997050/.

Daikoku, Ericko, et al. "Analysis of Morphology and Infectivity of Measles Virus Particles," Analysis of Morphology and Infectivity of Measles Virus Particles." *Bulletin of the Osaka Medical College*, 2007;53(2):107–14. https://www.semanticscholar.org/paper/Analysis-of-Morphology-and-Infectivity-of-Measles-Eriko-Daikoku/0b85babe55d54b0f58bca35f586852786f25b088.

Dalen et al., "The epidemic of the 20(th) century: coronary heart disease." *American Journal of Medicine*, 2014 Sep; 127(9):807–12. https://pubmed.ncbi.nlm.nih.gov/24811552/.

Dangor, Graison. "CDC's Six-Foot Social Distancing Rule Was 'Arbitrary,' Says Former FDA Commissioner." *Forbes*, September 19, 2021. https://www.forbes.com/sites/graisondangor/2021/09/19/cdcs-six-foot-social-distancing-rule-was-arbitrary-says-former-fda-commissioner/?sh=331efc39e8e6.

Daniel, Pete. *Toxic Drift: Pesticides and Health in the Post-World World War II South*. Baton Rouge: Louisiana State University Press, 2005.

Dennett, Preston. *The Healing Power of UFOs: 300 True Accounts of People Healed by Extraterrestrials*. Self-published, 2019.

Department of Health and Human Services. "FOI response: March 1, 2021." Fluoride Free Peel website, March 1, 2021. https://www.fluoridefreepeel.ca/wp-content/uploads/2021/03/CDC-March-1-2021-SARS-COV-2-Isolation-Response-Redacted.pdf.

Department of Health and Human Services. "FOI response: November 2, 2020." Fluoride Free Peel website, November 2, 2020. https://www.fluoridefreepeel.ca/wp-content/uploads/2020/11/USA-CDC-Virus-Isolation-Response-Scrubbed.pdf.

Department of Health and Human Services. "FOIA Request to CDC re: purification of the 'rabies virus.'" Fluoride Free Peel website, December 16, 2021. https://www.fluoridefreepeel.ca/wp-content/uploads/2021/12/CDC-rabies-PACKAGE-redacted.pdf.

Department of Health and Human Services. "FOIA Request to CDC re: 'smallpox virus' purification via any method." Fluoride Free Peel website, January 5, 2022. https://www.fluoridefreepeel.ca/wp-content/uploads/2022/01/CDC-smallpox-PACKAGE-redacted.pdf.

Department of Health and Human Services. "Re: FOIA Case Number: 50822, and HHS Appeal No.: 19-0083-AA." July 19, 2019. https://www.icandecide.org/wp-content/uploads/2020/08/20190719-HHS-Final-Response-IR0084-Appeal.pdf.

Dharan, Vandana, and Suja Aarattuthodi. "Rivers's Postulates Fulfilled for Blue Catfish Alloherpesvirus." *Frontiers in Environmental Microbiology,* September 2021; 7(3): 80–84. https://sciencepublishinggroup.com/journal/paperinfo?journalid=384&doi=10.11648/j.fem.20210703.12.

Division of Perceptual Studies. "Children Who Remember Previous Lives – Academic Publications." University of Virginia, Division of Perceptual Studies website, n.d. https://med.virginia.edu/perceptual-studies/publications/academic-publications/children-who-remember-previous-lives-academic-publications/.

D'Mello, J.P.F. (Ed.). *A Handbook of Environmental Toxicology: Human Disorders and Ecotoxicology.* Oxfordshire: CABI International, 2020.

Dolan, Richard. *The Alien Agendas: A Speculative Analysis of Those Visiting Earth.* Rochester, NY: Richard Dolan Press, 2020.

Dr. Andrew Kaufman. "Virus-Isolation: Is It Real? Andrew_Kaufman Responds to Jeremy Hammond." Odysee video, January 20, 2022. https://odysee.com/@DrAndrewKaufman:f/Virus_Isolation_Is_It_Real_Andrew_Kaufman_Responds_To_Jeremy-Hammond:9.

Dr. Sam Bailey. "Aluminium, Vaccines & Detox." Odysee video, January 23, 2023. https://odysee.com/@drsambailey:c/Aluminium-Vaccines-Detox:a?src=embed.

Dr. Sam Bailey. "Chickenpox Parties and Varicella Zoster Virus?" Dr. Sam Bailey's website, August 18, 2021. https://drsambailey.com/

resources/videos/viruses-unplugged/chickenpox-parties-and-varicella-zoster-virus/.

Dr. Sam Bailey. "Death Shot Doctors Stand Down." Odysee video, April 18, 2023. https://odysee.com/@drsambailey:c/Death-Shot-Doctors-Stand-Down:3?src=embed.

Dr. Sam Bailey. "Electron Microscopy and Unidentified 'Viral' Objects." Odysee video, February 16, 2022. https://drsambailey.com/resources/videos/covid-19/electron-microscopy-and-unidentified-viral-objects/.

Dr. Sam Bailey. "Fact-check: New Zealand can't find the 'SARS-CoV-2 virus.'" Dr. Sam Bailey website, February 12, 2022. https://drsambailey.com/fact-check-new-zealand-cant-find-the-sars-cov-2-virus/.

Dr. Sam Bailey. "5 Spectacular Fails From Germ Theory." Odysee website, September 12, 2023. https://odysee.com/@drsambailey:c/5-Spectacular-Fails-From-Germ-Theory:c?src=embed.

Dr. Sam Bailey. "The Follies of Peter McCullough." Odysee video, September, 17, 2023. https://odysee.com/@drsambailey:c/The-Follies-of-Peter-McCullough:4.

Dr. Sam Bailey. "Gain Of Function Garbage." Dr. Sam Bailey website, January 18, 2022. https://drsambailey.com/resources/videos/covid-19/gain-of-function-garbage//.

Dr. Sam Bailey. "Gain Of Function Gaslighting." Dr. Sam Bailey website, June 30, 2021. https://drsambailey.com/resources/videos/covid-19/gain-of-function-gaslighting/.

Dr. Sam Bailey, "Germ Theory vs Terrain Theory." Odysee video, May 25, 2021. https://odysee.com/@drsambailey:c/germ-theory-vs-terrain-theory:0?src=embed&t=348.702826.

Dr. Sam Bailey. "Koch's Postulates: Germ School Dropout." Dr. Sam Bailey website, September 8, 2021. https://drsambailey.com/resources/videos/germ-theory/kochs-postulates-germ-school-dropout/.

Dr. Sam Bailey. "Marvin vs. Virology: COVID Taken to Court." Odysee video, October 10, 2022. https://odysee.com/@drsambailey:c/Marvin-vs-Virology-COVID-Taken-To-Court:3.

Dr. Sam Bailey. "The Measles Myth." Odysee video, November 8, 2021. https://odysee.com/@drsambailey:c/themeaslesmyth:0.

Dr. Sam Bailey. "Peter McCullough's Shedding Stories." Dr. Sam Bailey website, June 10, 2023. https://drsambailey.com/resources/videos/vaccines/peter-mcculloughs-shedding-stories/.

Dr. Sam Bailey. "Runaway Virology—Marvin Win in Court." Odysee video, May 9, 2023. https://odysee.com/@drsambailey:c/Runaway-Virology-Marvin-Wins-In-Court:b?src=embed.

Dr. Sam Bailey. "Settling the Virus Debate" Statement." Dr. Sam Bailey website, https://drsambailey.com/resources/settling-the-virus-debate/.

Dr. Sam Bailey. "Stefan Lanka: "Virus, It's Time to Go." Odysee video, August 16, 2022. https://odysee.com/@drsambailey:c/Stefan-Lanka-Virus-Its-Time-To-Go:1?src=embed.

Dr. Sam Bailey. "TB: Cows, Lies & Koch-Ups." Odysee video, May 16, 2023. https://odysee.com/@drsambailey:c/TB-Cows-Lies-And-Koch-Ups:a.

Dr. Sam Bailey. "Tobacco Mosaic "Virus" – The beginning & end of virology." Dr. Sam Bailey website, April 5, 2022. https://drsambailey.com/resources/videos/viruses-unplugged/tobacco-mosaic-virus-the-beginning-and-end-of-virology/.

Dr. Sam Bailey. "The Truth About Antibiotics." Dr. Sam Bailey website, October 21, 2023. https://drsambailey.com/resources/videos/germ-theory/the-truth-about-antibiotics/.

Dr. Sam Bailey. "'Viruses' – Baileys, Cowan & Kaufman Respond to Del Bigtree." September 3, 2022. https://odysee.com/@drsambailey:c/Viruses-Baileys-Cowan-Kaufman-Respond-To-Del-Bigtree:b.

Dr. Sam Bailey. "What about Rabies?" Odysee video, August 9, 2022. https://odysee.com/@drsambailey:c/What-About-Rabies:a.

Dr. Sam Bailey. "What Happened to SARS-1?" Dr. Sam Bailey, January 26, 2021. https://odysee.com/@drsambailey:c/what-happened-to-sars-1:8.

Dr. Sam Bailey. "What We Weren't Taught About Hepatitis." Odysee video, June 6, 2023. https://odysee.com/@drsambailey:c/What-We-Weren't-Taught-About-Hepatitis:4.

Dr. Sam Bailey. "What We Weren't Taught About Herpes." Odysee video, June 7, 2022. https://odysee.com/@drsambailey:c/What-We-Weren't-Taught-About-Herpes:3?src=embed.

Chen, Jiaci et al. "Review on Strategies and Technologies for Exosome Isolation and Purification." *Front. Bioeng. Biotechnol.* 2022, Vol. 9, https://www.frontiersin.org/articles/10.3389/fbioe.2021.811971/full.

Dr. Tom Cowan. "A LOOK AT MALARIA – WEBINAR FROM JULY 12TH, 2023." Bitchute video, July 12, 2023. https://www.bitchute.com/video/SvHsnKFkJH4O/?list=notifications&randomize=false.

Dr. Tom Cowan. "Discussing the actual origin of the lab leak theory-Webinar from 10/18/23." Rumble video, October 18, 2023. https://rumble.com/v3q956g-discussing-the-actual-origin-of-the-lab-leak-theory-webinar-from-101823.html?mref=6zof&mc=dgip3&ep=2.

Dr. Tom Cowan. "HOW TO MAKE A POLIO VACCINE + A REBUTTAL- WEBINAR FROM AUGUST 30TH, 2023." Bitchute video, August 30, 2023. https://www.bitchute.com/video/WaPyKutv4Oz9/.

Dr. Tom Cowan. "MY DISCUSSION WITH STEFAN LANKA ABOUT VIROLOGY." Bitchute video, March 25, 2021. https://www.bitchute.com/video/oBJOwKpgtDqX/.

Dr. Tom Cowan. "NUCLEAR ATOM & RESPONSE TO VERNON COLEMAN 9/6/23 WEBINAR." Bitchute video, September 6, 2023. https://www.bitchute.com/video/BC25ikU2sTKt/.

Dr. Tom Cowan. "WEBINAR WITH DR. MARK BAILEY ON THE HART GROUP: OCTOBER 11, 2023." Bitchute video, October 11, 2023. https://www.bitchute.com/video/lAJp8FwPrMSi/.

Ducharme, Robert. "COLUMNS Latest changes to Condominium Act are significant." *Foster's Daily Democrat*, September 2, 2018. https://www.fosters.com/story/business/columns/2018/09/02/latest-changes-to-condominium-act-are-significant/10864840007/.

Duesberg, Peter. *Inventing the AIDS Virus*. Washington, DC: Regnery Publishing, 1996.

Duffy, Thomas. "The Flexner Report—100 Years Later." *Yale J Biol Med.* 2011 Sep;84(3):269–76. https://www.ncbi.nlm.nih.gov/pmc/articles/PMC3178858/.

EarthNewspaper.com. "ANTIVIRAL OR NONSENSE BY DR. THOMAS COWAN." Bitchute video, April 2, 2022. https://www.bitchute.com/video/5NtlfxqCBzw7/.

Egerton, R. F., *Physical Principles of Electron Microscopy.* Switzerland: Springer International Publishing, 2016.

Enders, John F., and Thomas C. Peebles. "Propagation in Tissue Cultures of Cytopathogenic Agents from Patients with Measles." *Proc Soc Exp Biol Med,* 1954 Jun;86(2):277–86.

The End of COVID. N.d. https://theendofcovid.com/.

Engdahl, William. "Toxicology vs. Virology: Rockefeller Institute and the Criminal Polio Fraud." William Engdahl's website, July 12, 2022. http://williamengdahl.com/englishNEO12July2022.php.

Engelbrecht, Torsten, Claus Köhnlein, and Samantha Bailey. *Virus Mania* (3rd edition). 2021. First published in 2007 by Trafford Publishing.

Epstein, Steven. *Impure Science: AIDS, Activism, and the Politics of Knowledge.* Berkeley: University of California Press, 1996.

ESR. "Official Information Act Request: FOIA: SARS-COV-2 Proof of Existence." Letter dated July 19, 2022. https://www.fluoridefreepeel.ca/wp-content/uploads/2022/08/NZ-ESR-No-Proof-Of-Existence.pdf.

ESR. "Official Information Act Request: SARS-COV-2 Proof of Causation," August 17, 2022. https://www.fluoridefreepeel.ca/wp-content/uploads/2022/09/2022-08-29-ESR-SARS-COV-2-Proof-of-Causation-Redacted.pdf.

Exley, Christopher. "The toxicity of aluminum in humans." *Morphologie,* June 2016; 100(329), 51–55. https://www.sciencedirect.com/science/article/abs/pii/S1286011516000023.

Facher, Lev. "More than two-thirds of Congress cashed a pharma campaign check in 2020, new STAT analysis shows." Prescription Politics website, June 9, 2021. https://www.statnews.com/feature/prescription-politics/federal-full-data-set/.

Faith-Masterson, Serena. *I Am Serena*. Dream Magic Publications, 2020.

Farber, Celia. *Serious Adverse Events: An Uncensored History of AIDS*. White River Junction: Chelsea Green Publishing, 2006.

Fenton, Bruce, and Daniella Fenton. *Exogenesis: Hybrid Humans*. Newburyport, MA: New Page Books, 2020.

Find a Grave. "Dr Matthew Joseph Rodermund." Find a Grave website, n.d. https://www.findagrave.com/memorial/175430985/matthew-joseph-rodermund.

Firstenberg, Arthur. *The Invisible Rainbow: A History of Electricity*. White River Junction, VT: Chelsea Green Publishing: 2020.

Flexner, Abraham. *Medical Education in the United States and Canada*. New York: The Carnegie Foundation for the Advancement of Teaching, 1910.

Flexner, Simon, and Paul Lewis. "The Transmission of Acute Poliomyelitis to Monkeys." *JAMA*, 1909; 250(6).

Fluoride Free Peel. "Do health and science institutions have studies proving that bacteria CAUSE disease?" Fluoride Free Peel, n.d. https://www.fluoridefreepeel.ca/do-health-authorities-have-studies-proving-that-bacteria-cause-disease-lets-find-out-via-freedom-of-information/.

Fluoride Free Peel. "FOIs reveal that health/science institutions have no record of any 'virus' having been found in a host and isolated/purified. Because virology isn't a science." Fluoride Free Peel website, November 7, 2021. https://www.fluoridefreepeel.ca/fois-reveal-that-health-science-institutions-have-no-record-of-any-virus-having-been-isolated-purified-virology-isnt-a-science/.

Foley, Katherine Ellen. "Trust issues deepen as yet another FDA commissioner joins the pharmaceutical industry," July 1, 2019. https://qz.com/1656529/yet-another-fda-commissioner-joins-the-pharmaceutical-industry.

Fouchier, Ron et al. "Koch's postulates fulfilled for SARS virus." *Nature* 423, 240 (2003). https://www.nature.com/articles/423240a/.

Friese, Thomas. "Preface" to *The Forest Passage* by Ernst Jünger. Candor: Telos Press Publishing, 2013.

Galeano, Eduardo. *Open Veins of Latin America*. New York: Monthly Review Press, 1997.

Gallagher, Richard. *Demonic Foes*. New York: HarperOne, 2022.

Gear, JH. "Nonpolio causes of polio-like paralytic syndromes." *Rev Infect Dis*, 1984 May-Jun:6 Suppl 2:S379-84. https://pubmed.ncbi.nlm.nih.gov/6740077/.

Geison, Gerald. *The Private Science of Louis Pasteur*. Princeton: Princeton University Press, 1995.

Gladstone, William. *Miracle Soul Healer*. Dallas: BenBella Books, 2014.

The Global Consciousness Project. "Formal Results: Testing the GCP Hypothesis." Global Consciousness Project website, n.d. globalmind.org/results.html.

Gober, Mark. *An End to Upside Down Contact: UFOs, Aliens, and Spirits—and Why Their Ongoing Interaction with Human Civilization Matters*. Cardiff-by-the-Sea, CA: Waterside Productions, 2022.

Gober, Mark. *An End to Upside Down Liberty: Turning Traditional Political Thinking on Its Head to Break Free from Enslavement*. Cardiff-by-the-Sea, CA: Waterside Productions, 2021.

Gober, Mark. *An End to Upside Down Living: Reorienting Our Consciousness to Live Better and Save the Human Species*. Cardiff-by-the-Sea, CA: Waterside Productions, 2020.

Gober, Mark. *An End to Upside Down Thinking: Dispelling the Myth That the Brain Produces Consciousness, and the Implications for Everyday Life*. Cardiff-by-the-Sea, CA: Waterside Publishing, 2018.

Gober, Mark. *An End to the Upside Down Reset: The Leftist Vision for Society Under the Great Reset—and How It Can Fool Caring People into Supporting Harmful Causes*. Cardiff-by-the-Sea, CA: Waterside Productions, 2023.

Gober, Mark, and Blue Duck Media. *Where Is My Mind?* Podcast (Eps. 1 through 8). June–September 2019.

Goel, Vritti Rashi. "Facebook widens ban on vaccine misinformation." CBS News, February 8, 2021. https://www.cbsnews.com/news/

facebook-widens-ban-on-vaccine-misinformation-to-include-anti-vaccination-conspiracy-theories/.

GoodTherapy. "Family Constellations." GoodTherapy website, n.d. https://www.goodtherapy.org/learn-about-therapy/types/family-constellations.

Gøtzcshe, Peter. *Deadly Medicines and Organized Crime: How Big pharma has corrupted healthcare*. Boca Raton: CRC Press, 2017.

Grafe, Alfred. *A History of Experimental Virology*. Berlin: Springer Verlag, 1991.

Greene, Brian. *The Fabric of the Cosmos: Space, Time, and the Texture of Reality*. New York: A.A. Knopf, 2004.

Greyson, Bruce. *After: A Doctor Explores What Near-Death Experiences Reveal about Life and Beyond*. New York: Saint Martin's Essentials, 2021.

Greyson, Bruce. "Seeing Dead People Not Known to Have Died: "Peak in Darien" Experiences." *Anthropology and Humanism*, November 21, 2010. https://anthrosource.onlinelibrary.wiley.com/doi/abs/10.1111/j.1548-1409.2010.01064.x.

Greyson, Bruce et al. "Recent Report of Electroencephalogram of a Dying Human Brain." Invited commentary, 2022. https://www.iands.org/images/stories/pdf_downloads/Greyson_et_al-2022-Commentary-on-Report-of-EEG-in-a-Dying-Human-Brain.pdf.

GSK. "ENERGIX-B" package insert. n.d., https://www.fda.gov/media/119403/download.

Gussak et al. *Iatrogenicity: Causes and Consequences of Iatrogenesis in Cardiovascular Medicine*. New Brunswick, NJ: Rutgers University Press, 2015.

Haberer, Rod. *Healer: The Jerry Wills Story*. Rod Haberer, 2012.

Hammond, Jeremy. "Cowan and Haberland Illuminate the Dogma of Virus Denialism." Jeremy R. Hammond website, November 9, 2022. https://www.jeremyrhammond.com/2022/11/09/study-finds-42-false-discovery-rate-for-sars-cov-2-pcr-tests/.

HART. "Why HART uses the virus model." HART's website, October 4, 2023. https://www.hartgroup.org/virus-model/.

Harvard Health Publishing. "Blue light has a dark side." Harvard Medical School website, July 7, 2020. https://www.health.harvard.edu/staying-healthy/blue-light-has-a-dark-side.

Harvard Pilgrim Health Care, Inc. "Electronic Support for Public Health–Vaccine Adverse Event Reporting System (ESP: VAERS)." 2007–2010. https://censored.vaxcalc.org/wp-content/uploads/2019/06/r18hs017045-lazarus-final-report-2011.pdf.

Hawden, Walter. "Sanitation v. Vaccination: The Origin of Smallpox." *Truth*, January 17, 1923. https://www.soilandhealth.org/wp-content/uploads/GoodBooks/Hadwin-%20Table%20of%20Contents.pdf.

Hawkins, David. *Healing and Recovery*. Alexandria, Australia: Hay House, 2009.

Hawkins, David. *Letting Go: The Pathway of Surrender*. Alexandria, Australia: Hay House, 2014.

Healing Powers with Laura Powers. "Mira Kelley and Past Lives." April 19, 2016. https://music.amazon.co.uk/podcasts/5698afd2-031d-400b-853f-b51d96770612/episodes/3496420b-cbf3-496a-9cb4-53bd278bbd59/healing-powers-podcast-mira-kelley-and-past-lives.

Heckenlively, Kent. *Inoculated: How Science Lost Its Soul in Autism*. Cardiff-by-the-Sea, CA: Waterfront Press, 2016.

Helfrich-Förster, C. et al. "Women temporarily synchronize their menstrual cycles with the luminance and gravimetric cycles of the Moon." *Sci Adv*, January 27, 2021;7(5). https://pubmed.ncbi.nlm.nih.gov/33571128/.

Hensley, Laura. "Big pharma pours millions into medical schools — here's how it can impact education." *Global News*, August 12, 2019. https://globalnews.ca/news/5738386/canadian-medical-school-funding/.

Hess, Alfred. "Need of Further Research on the Transmissibility of Measles and Varicella." *JAMA*, 1919;73(16):1232. https://jamanetwork.com/journals/jama/article-abstract/222413?resultClick=1.

Hezakya Newz & Films. "1988 THROWBACK: 'DR FAUCI SAYS AZT AIDS DRUG IS SAFE AND EFFECTIVE.'"

YouTube video, June 17, 2021. https://www.youtube.com/watch?v=fKWwEkBZjhM.

Hillman, Harold. *The Case for New Paradigms in Cell Biology and Neurobiology*. Lewiston, NY: The Edwin Mellen Press, 1991.

History. "Spanish Flu." *History*, May 10, 2023. https://www.history.com/topics/world-war-i/1918-flu-pandemic.

Hodge, John. *The Vaccine Superstition*. Niagara Falls, 1902.

Horikami, S. M., and S. A. Moyer. "Structure, transcription, and replication of measles virus." *Curr Top Microbiol Immunol*, 1995;191:35-50. https://pubmed.ncbi.nlm.nih.gov/7789161/.

Housatonic.Live. "Ep 200.1: Dr. Mark Bailey (author of "A Farewell to Virology") questions pathogenic viruses." Odysee video, February 13, 2023. https://odysee.com/@Housatonic:0/539-ep-200-1:3.

houseofnumbers. "Prof. Luc Montagnier's Extended House of Numbers Interview." YouTube video, April 23, 2011. https://www.youtube.com/watch?v=PyPq-waF-h4.

HRSA, "Data and Statistics." September 1, 2023. https://www.hrsa.gov/sites/default/files/hrsa/vicp/vicp-stats-09-01-23.pdf.

Huang, Yanzhong. "THE SARS EPIDEMIC AND ITS AFTERMATH IN CHINA: A POLITICAL PERSPECTIVE." National Library of Medicine website, 2004. https://www.ncbi.nlm.nih.gov/books/NBK92479/.

Hume, Ethel. *Béchamp or Pasteur?: A Lost Chapter in the History of Biology*. CreateSpace Independent Publishing Platform, 2011.

Humphries, Suzanne. *Rising from the Dead*. Suzanne Humphries, MD, 2016.

Humphries, Suzanne, and Roman Bystrianyk. *Dissolving Illusions: Disease, Vaccines, and Forgotten History*. Suzanne Humphries, MD, and Roman Bystrianyk, 2015.

The Infectious Myth. "The Infectious Myth – Thomas Cowan on COVID-19 and Germ Theory." June 2, 2020. https://podcasts.apple.com/us/podcast/the-infectious-myth/id829019119?i=1000476566837.

Informed Consent Action Network. "NIH Concedes It Has No Studies Assessing The Safety Of Injecting Aluminum Adjuvants."

ICANdecide website, August 2020. https://www.icandecide.org/ican_government/nih-concedes-it-has-no-studies-assessing-the-safety-of-injecting-aluminum-adjuvants/.

INSTITUTE FOR AUTISM SCIENCE AND THE INFORMED CONSENT ACTION NETWORK vs. CENTERS FOR DISEASE CONTROL AND PREVENTION, Complaint for Case 1:19-cv-11947. Filed December 31, 2019. https://www.icandecide.org/wp-content/uploads/2020/03/001-COMPLAINT-against-Centers-for-Disease-Control-and-Prevention.pdf.

The Internet Encyclopedia of Mind. "The Hard Problem of Consciousness," The Internet Encyclopedia of Mind website, n.d. https://iep.utm.edu/hard-problem-of-conciousness/.

"Interview with Max Planck." *The Observer*, January 25, 1931.

Jain, Shamini. *Healing Ourselves: Biofield Science and the Future of Health.* Boulder, CO: Sounds True, 2021.

Jain, Shamini. LinkedIn post, August 2023. https://www.linkedin.com/feed/update/urn:li:activity:7101565388223565824/.

Janssen, Volker. "When Polio Triggered Fear and Panic Among Parents in the 1950s." *History*, September 11, 2023. https://www.history.com/news/polio-fear-post-wwii-era.

JeffMara Podcast. "Man Struck By Lighting; DIED & Was Told The Future (NDE) | Dannion Brinkley." YouTube video, August 20, 2023. https://youtu.be/l1HasR5er3c.

jerrywills. "Jerry Wills on FOX 2006." YouTube video, June 13, 2007. https://www.youtube.com/watch?v=J0e7uUPtALs.

Johns Hopkins Bloomberg School of Public Health. "Spending on Consumer Advertising for Top-Selling Prescription Drugs in U.S. Favors Those With Low Added Benefit." Johns Hopkins Bloomberg School of Public Health website, February 7, 2023. https://publichealth.jhu.edu/2023/spending-on-consumer-advertising-for-top-selling-prescription-drugs-in-us-favors-those-with-low-added-benefit.

Jordan, Miriam. "In Texas, a Quarantine Camp for Migrants With Covid-19." *New York Times*, August 12, 2021. https://www.nytimes.com/2021/08/12/us/coronavirus-migrants-border-covid.html.

Kadagian, DJ. *Crossover Experience: Life-After-Death; A New Perspective*. Four Seasons Productions, 2022.

Kastrup, Bernardo. *Brief Peeks Beyond: Critical Essays on Metaphysics, Neuroscience, Free Will, Skepticism, and Culture*. Winchester, UK: Iff, 2015.

Kastrup, Bernardo. *The Idea of the World: A Multi-Disciplinary Argument for the Mental Nature of Reality*. Hampshire, UK: Iff, 2019.

Kastrup, Bernardo. *More Than Allegory: On Religious Myth, Truth and Belief*. Winchester, UK: John Hunt 2016.

Kastrup, Bernardo. "Transcending the Brain: At Least Some Cases of Physical Damage Are Associated with Enriched Consciousness or Cognitive Skill." *Scientific American* blog, March 29, 2017. https://blogs.scientificamerican.com/guest-blog/transcending-the-brain/.

Kastrup, Bernardo. *Why Materialism Is Baloney: How True Skeptics Know There Is No Death and Fathom Answers to Life, the Universe and Everything*. Winchester, UK: Iff, 2014.

Kastrup, Bernardo et al. "Disorder Explain Life, the Universe and Everything?" *Scientific American*, June 18, 2018. https://blogs.scientificamerican.com/observations/could-multiple-personality-disorder-explain-life-the-universe-and-everything/.

Kastrup, Bernardo, and Edward Kelly. "Misreporting and Confirmation Bias in Psychedelic Research." *Scientific American*, September 3, 2018. https://blogs.scientificamerican.com/observations/misreporting-and-confirmation-bias-in-psychedelic-research/.

Kelly, Edward. "Best way forward or unnecessary detour? A review of 'Dual-Aspect Monism and the Deep Structure of Meaning.'" Essentia Foundation website, August 27, 2023. https://www.essentiafoundation.org/best-way-forward-or-unnecessary-detour-a-review-of-dual-aspect-monism-and-the-deep-structure-of-meaning/reading/.

Kennedy Jr., Robert. *The Real Anthony Fauci: Bill Gates, Big Pharma, and the Global War on Democracy and Public Health*. New York: Skyhorse Publishing, 2021.

Kennedy Jr., Robert. *Thimerosal: Let the Science Speak*. New York: Skyhorse Publishing, 2015.

Kennedy Jr., Robert, and Brian Hooker. *Vax-Unvax: Let the Science Speak*. New York: Skyhorse Publishing 2023.

Killingley, Ben et al. "Use of a Human Influenza Challenge Model to Assess Person-to-Person Transmission: Proof-of Concept Study." *The Journal of Infectious Diseases*, January 2012; 205(1), 35–43. https://academic.oup.com/jid/article/205/1/35/876311.

Kimble, Lindsay. "Pamela Anderson Announces She's Cured of Hepatitis C – See the Racy Photo She Posted to Celebrate." *People*, November 9, 2015. https://people.com/celebrity/pamela-anderson-is-cured-of-hep-c-see-the-photo-she-posted-to-celebrate/.

Kiuken, Thijs et al. "Newly discovered coronavirus as the primary cause of severe acute respiratory syndrome." *The Lancet*, July 2003; 362 (9380): 263-270. https://www.thelancet.com/journals/lancet/article/PIIS0140-6736(03)13967-0/fulltext.

Koster, John. "SMALLPOX BLANKETS: MYTH OR MASSACRE?" HISTORYNET website, August 15, 2017. https://www.historynet.com/smallpox-in-the-blankets/.

Lanka, Stefan. "The Misconception called 'Virus.'" Internet Archive, November 16, 2020. https://archive.org/details/paper-virus-lanka-002/mode/2up.

Lauritsen, John. *Poison by Prescription: The AZT Story*. New York: ASKLEPIOS/Pagan Press, 1990.

Ledford, Heidi. "Luc Montagnier (1932–2022)." *Nature*, March 4, 2022. https://www.nature.com/articles/d41586-022-00653-y.

Legal Information Institute. "42 U.S. Code § 300aa–11 – Petitions for compensation." Cornell Law School, n.d. https://www.law.cornell.edu/uscode/text/42/300aa-11.

Lester, Dawn, and David Parker. *What Really Makes You Ill? Why Everything You Thought You Knew About Disease Is Wrong*. Dawn Lester and David Parker, 2019.

Lipton, Bruce. *The Biology of Belief: Unleashing the Power of Consciousness, Matter & Miracles*. Carlsbad, CA: Hay House, 2015.

Lipton, Bruce. "THINK Beyond Your Genes – September 2021." Bruce Lipton, PhD's website, September 30, 2021. https://www.brucelipton.com/think-beyond-your-genes-september-2021/.

Long, Jeffrey, with Paul Perry. *God and the Afterlife: The Groundbreaking New Evidence for God and Near-Death Experience*. New York: HarperCollins, 2016.

Lund, G.A. et al. "The Molecular Length of Measles Virus RNA and the Structural Organization of Measles Nucleocapsids." *Journal of General Virology*, September 1984; 65(9):1535–42. https://www.microbiologyresearch.org/content/journal/jgv/10.1099/0022-1317-65-9-1535.

Mack, John. *Abduction: Human Encounters with Aliens*. New York: Macmillan Publishing Company, 1994.

Mack, John E. "The Believer: Ralph Blumenthal and Leslie Kean on Alien Encounters." YouTube video, May 23, 2021. https://www.youtube.com/watch?v=BMOBoaSqegc.

Mack, John. *Passport to the Cosmos: Human Transformation and Alien Encounters*. Guildford, UK: White Crow Books, 2011.

Mack, John. "STUDYING INTRUSIONS FROM THE SUBTLE REALM: HOW CAN WE DEEPEN OUR KNOWLEDGE." In *Making Contact: Preparing for the New Realities of Extraterrestrial Existence*. New York: St. Martin's Publishing Group, 2021.

Makary, Martin and Michael Daniel. "Medical error-the third leading cause of death in the US." *BMJ* May 2016, 353:i2139. https://pubmed.ncbi.nlm.nih.gov/27143499/.

Manek, Nish. "Do women's periods really sync up?" *BBC Science Focus*, May 11, 2021. https://www.sciencefocus.com/the-human-body/do-periods-sync.

Maready, Forrest. *The Moth in the Iron Lung*. Forrest Maready, 2018.

Markolin, Caroline. "THE FIVE BIOLOGICAL LAWS OF THE NEW MEDICINE." Learning GNM website, n.d. https://learninggnm.com/SBS/documents/five_laws.html.

Markolin, Caroline. "Measles Virus Put to the Test." Learning GNM website, n.d. https://learninggnm.com/SBS/documents/Lanka_Bardens_Trial_E.pdf.

Matherne, Bobby. "The Fall of the Spirits of Darkness, GA#177 14 Lectures in Dornach in 1917 by Rudolf Steiner." http://www.doyletics.com/arj/falldark.pdf.

Matlock, James. *Signs of Reincarnation: Exploring Beliefs, Cases, and Theory*. London: Rowman & Littlefield, 2019.

Mayo Clinic. "E. coli." Mayo Clinic website, n.d. https://www.mayoclinic.org/diseases-conditions/e-coli/symptoms-causes/syc-20372058.

Mayo Clinic. "Polio." Mayo Clinic website, n.d. https://www.mayoclinic.org/diseases-conditions/history-disease-outbreaks-vaccine-timeline/polio.

McBean, Eleanor. *The Poisoned Needle: Suppressed Facts about Vaccination*. Eleanor McBean, 1957.

McBean, Eleanor. *Swine Flu Expose*. 1977, http://whale.to/vaccine/sf1.html.

McCraty, Rollin. *Science of the Heart*. Boulder Creek, CO: HeartMath Institute, 2015.

McKusick, Eileen. *Electric Body, Electric Health*. New York: St. Martin's Publishing, 2021.

McMains, Vanessa. "Johns Hopkins study suggests medical errors are third-leading cause of death in U.S." Johns Hopkins University website, May 3, 2016. https://hub.jhu.edu/2016/05/03/medical-errors-third-leading-cause-of-death/.

Mercola, Joseph. "EMF Pollution and Chronic Disease — What's the Connection?" Children's Health Defense website, December 16, 2022. https://childrenshealthdefense.org/defender/emf-pollution-chronic-disease-cola/.

Merriam-Webster. "isolate." *Merriam-Webster*, n.d. https://www.merriam-webster.com/dictionary/isolate.

MES Truth. "2009 HIV/AIDS Documentary: House of Numbers – Anatomy of an Epidemic." YouTube video, April 4, 2021. https://www.youtube.com/watch?v=lvDqjXTByF4.

Microscope Master. "What is Cryo-Electron Microscopy?" Microscope Master website, n.d., https://www.microscopemaster.com/cryo-electron-microscopy.html.

Morgan, Ewan. "The Physician Who Presaged the Germ Theory of Disease Nearly 500 Years Ago." *Scientific American*, January 22, 2021. https://www.scientificamerican.com/article/the-physician-who-presaged-the-germ-theory-of-disease-nearly-500-years-ago/.

Moorjani, Anita. "The Day My Life Changed: February 2, 2006." Anita Moorjani webpage, n.d. http://anitamoorjani.com/about-anita/near-death-experience-description/.

Moorjani, Anita. *Dying to Be Me: My Journey from Cancer, to Near Death, to True Healing*. New Delhi, India: Hay House, 2015.

Mossbridge, Julia. "Physiological Activity That Seems to Anticipate Future Events." In *Evidence for Psi: Thirteen Empirical Research Reports*, edited by Damien Broderick and Ben Goertzel. Jefferson, NC: McFarland, 2015.

Mossbridge J., P. Tressoldi, and J. Utts. "Predictive Physiological Anticipation Preceding Seemingly Unpredictable Stimuli: A Meta-Analysis." *Frontiers in Psychology* 3 (2012): 390. https://www.frontiersin.org/articles/10.3389/fpsyg.2012.00390/full.

Mossbridge, Julia et al. "Predicting the Unpredictable: Critical Analysis and Practical Implications of Predictive Anticipatory Activity." *Frontiers in Human Neuroscience*, 8 (2014): 146. https://www.ncbi.nlm.nih.gov/pmc/articles/PMC3971164/.

Mullis, Kary. *Dancing Naked in the Mind Field*. New York: Pantheon Books, 1998.

Nakai, Masuyo, and David Imagawa, "Electron Microscopy of Measles Virus Replication." *J Virol*. 1969 Feb; 3(2): 187–197. https://www.ncbi.nlm.nih.gov/pmc/articles/PMC375751/.

National Cancer Institute. "National Cancer Act of 1971." National Cancer Institute website, n.d. https://dtp.cancer.gov/timeline/flash/milestones/M4_Nixon.htm.

National Institute of Environmental Health Sciences. "Formaldehyde." National Institute of Environmental Health Sciences website, n.d. https://www.niehs.nih.gov/health/topics/agents/formaldehyde/index.cfm.

Nature. "Submission guidelines." *Nature* website, n.d. https://www.nature.com/srep/author-instructions/submission-guidelines#methods.

Nelson, R. D. et al. "Correlations of Continuous Random Data With Major World Events." *Foundations of Physics Letters* 15 (2002): 537–50.

New York Times, "Dr. Rodermund Escapes. Man Who Caused Smallpox Scare Gets Away from Appleton." *New York Times*, January 28, 1901. https://timesmachine.nytimes.com/timesmachine/1901/01/28/102439229.html?pageNumber=8.

NIH. "The Discovery of the Double Helix, 1951-1953." NIH Library of Medicine website, n.d. https://profiles.nlm.nih.gov/spotlight/sc/feature/doublehelix.

Niu, Qiao. "Overview of the Relationship Between Aluminum Exposure and Health of Human Being." *Adv Exp Med Biol.* 2018;1091:1-31. https://pubmed.ncbi.nlm.nih.gov/30315446/.

NobelPrize.org. "The Nobel Prize in Physiology or Medicine 1969." NobelPrize.org, September 23, 2023. https://www.nobelprize.org/prizes/medicine/1969/summary/.

Null et al. *Death by Medicine*. Edinburg: Axios Press, 2011.

Official Church of the FSM. https://www.spaghettimonster.org/.

Olmsted, Dan, and Mark Blaxill. *The Age of Autism: Mercury, Medicine, and a Man-Made Epidemic*. New York: Thomas Dunne Books, 2010.

Olmsted, Dan, and Mark Blaxill. *Denial: How Refusing to Face the Facts about Our Autism Epidemic Hurts Children, Families, and Our Future*. New York: Skyhorse Publishing, 2017.

O'Neill, Natalie. "Fauci says attacks on him are 'attacks on science.'" *New York Post*, June 9, 2021. https://nypost.com/2021/06/09/fauci-says-attacks-on-him-are-attacks-on-science/.

Padian et al. "Heterosexual Transmission of Human Immunodeficiency Virus (HIV) in Northern California: Results from a Ten-year Study." *American Journal of Epidemiology*, August 1997; 146(4): 350–57. https://academic.oup.com/aje/article/146/4/350/60711?login=false.

Passon, Oliver. "Kelvin's Clouds." *Am. J. Phys.*, November 2021; 89(11): 1037–41. https://pubs.aip.org/aapt/ajp/article-abstract/89/11/1037/859801/Kelvin-s-clouds?redirectedFrom=fulltext.

Papadopulos-Eleopulos, E. et al. "HIV—A virus like no other." Perth Group website, July 12, 2017. http://www.theperthgroup.com/HIV/TPGVirusLikeNoOther.pdf.

Patel, Girijesh Kumar et al. "Comparative analysis of exosome isolation methods using culture supernatant for optimum yield, purity and downstream applications." *Sci Rep* 9, 5335 (2019). https://doi.org/10.1038/s41598-019-41800-2.

Pearsall, Paul. *The Heart's Code: Tapping the Wisdom and Power of Our Heart Energy; The New Findings About Cellular Memories and Their Role in the Mind, Body, Spirit Connection.* New York: Broadway, 1999.

Peer, RF, and Shabir, N. "Iatrogenesis: A review on nature, extent, and distribution of healthcare hazards." *J Family Med Prim Care.* 2018 Mar-Apr;7(2):309-314. https://www.ncbi.nlm.nih.gov/pmc/articles/PMC6060929/.

Perry, Mark. "Michael Crichton Explains Why There Is 'No Such Thing as Consensus Science.'" *AEI*, December 15, 2019. https://www.aei.org/carpe-diem/michael-crichton-explains-why-there-is-no-such-thing-as-consensus-science/.

Plescia, Marissa. "Are We Prepared for the Next Pandemic? Anthony Fauci Weighs In at AHIP." *MedCityNews*, June 14, 2023. https://medcitynews.com/2023/06/fauci-covid-pandemic-vaccines-public-health/.

Pollack, Gerald. *The Fourth Phase of Water: Beyond Solid Liquid Vapor.* Seattle: Ebner & Sons Publishers, 2013.

Princeton Engineering Anomalies Research. N.d. http://pearlab.icrl.org/.

Pruitt-Young, Sharon. "YouTube Is Banning All Content That Spreads Vaccine Misinformation." NPR, September 29, 2021. https://www.npr.org/2021/09/29/1041493544/youtube-vaccine-misinformation-ban.

Public Health Agency of Canada. "Response to Christine Massey 20 December, 2021." Fluoride Free Peel website, December 20, 2021. https://www.fluoridefreepeel.ca/wp-content/uploads/2022/01/PHAC-ANY-virus-PACKAGE-redacted.pdf.

Question Everything, "Dr Robert Willner Injects 'HIV' into himself on TV." YouTube video, March 25, 2011. https://www.youtube.com/watch?v=tQCKb1JV-4A.

Radin, Dean. *The Conscious Universe: The Scientific Truth of Psychic Phenomena*. New York: HarperEdge, 1997.

Radin, Dean. *Entangled Minds Extrasensory Experiences in a Quantum Reality*. New York: Paraview, 2006.

Radin, Dean. "Publications." Dean Radin website, n.d. https://www.deanradin.com/publications.

Radin, Dean. *Real Magic: Ancient Wisdom, Modern Science, and a Guide to the Secret Power of the Universe*. New York: Harmony, 2018.

Radin, Dean. *Supernormal: Science, Yoga, and the Evidence for Extraordinary Psychic Abilities*. New York: Random House, 2013.

Radin, Dean et al. "Re-Examining Psychokinesis: Commentary on the Bösch, Steinkamp, and Boller Meta-Analysis." *Psychological Bulletin* 132 (2006): 529–32.

Rai, Alin et al. "A Protocol for Isolation, Purification, Characterization, and Functional Dissection of Exosomes." *Methods Mol Biol.* 2261 (2021):105–49.

Rasnick, David. "Rapid Response: Sex has nothing to do with AIDS." *BMJ*, January 18, 2003. https://www.bmj.com/rapid-response/2011/10/29/sex-has-nothing-do-aids.

Raj, Gopal. "Polio free does not mean paralysis free." *The Hindu*, January 3, 2013. https://www.thehindu.com/opinion/lead/polio-free-does-not-mean-paralysis-free/article4266043.ece.

Rappuoli, Rino. "1885, the first rabies vaccination in humans." *PNAS*, August 26, 2014. https://www.pnas.org/doi/10.1073/pnas.1414226111.

Rasmussen Reports. "COVID-19: Democratic Voters Support Harsh Measures Against Unvaccinated." Rassmussen Reports website, January 13, 2022. https://www.rasmussenreports.com/public_content/politics/partner_surveys/jan_2022/covid_19_democratic_voters_support_harsh_measures_against_unvaccinated.

Ravindran et al. "A Non-enveloped Virus Hijacks Host Disaggregation Machinery to Translocate across the Endoplasmic

Reticulum Membrane." *PLOS Pathogens*, August 15, 2015. https://journals.plos.org/plospathogens/article?id=10.1371/journal.ppat.1005086.

Rawat, KS, and Titus Rivas. *Reincarnation as a Scientific Concept: Scholarly Evidence for Past Lives*. United Kingdom: White Crow Books, 2021.

Rawlette, Sharon Hewitt. "Does an Afterlife Obviously Exist?" *Psychology Today*, April 29, 2022. https://www.psychologytoday.com/gb/blog/mysteries-consciousness/202204/does-afterlife-obviously-exist.

Raypole, Crystal. "What Is the Nocebo Effect?" Heathline website, February 25, 2019. https://www.healthline.com/health/nocebo-effect#how-it-works.

Reclamation Radio with Kelly Brogan, MD. "Why German New Medicine with Dr. Melissa Sell." July 25, 2023. https://podcasts.apple.com/us/podcast/reclamation-radio-with-kelly-brogan-md/id1663947298?i=1000622254539.

Relman, Arnold. "The New Medical-Industrial Complex." *N Engl J Med* 1980; 303:963-970.

The Ring of Fire. "Big Pharma Owns Corporate Media, and It's Killing People." YouTube video, July 26, 2018. https://www.youtube.com/watch?v=q3lviBkaEUc.

Rivas, Titas, Anny Dirven, and Rudolf H. Smit. *The Self Does Not Die: Verified Paranormal Phenomena from Near-Death Experiences*. Durham: IANDS Publications, 2016.

Roingeard, Philippe. "Viral detection by electron microscopy: past, present and future," *Biol Cell*, 2008 Aug; 100(8): 491–501. https://www.ncbi.nlm.nih.gov/pmc/articles/PMC7161876/.

Rosenau, Milton. "Experiments to Determine Mode of Spread of Influenza." *JAMA*, 1919;73(5):311–13. https://jamanetwork.com/journals/jama/article-abstract/221687.

Rosenau, Milton. "Experiments upon volunteers to determine the cause and mode of spread of influenza, Boston, November and December, 1918." *Treasury Department: United States Public Health Service*, February, 1921, 5–41. https://quod.lib.umich.edu/cgi/t/text/idx/f/flu/3750flu.0016.573/1/--experiments-upon-volunteers-to-determine-the-cause-and-mode?rgn=subject; view=image;q1=virology.

Ross, Colin A. *The C.I.A. Doctors: Human Rights Violations by American Psychiatrists*. Richardson: Manitou Communications, Inc., 2006.

Sanexa, Vivek. "New study shared by NIH suggests N95 Covid masks create dangerous of level toxic compounds linked seizures, cancer." *BPR: Business & Politics*, August 27, 2023. https://www.bizpacreview.com/2023/08/27/new-study-shared-by-nih-suggests-n95-covid-masks-create-dangerous-of-level-toxic-compounds-linked-seizures-cancer-1390631/.

Schlitz, Marilyn. "Spontaneous Remission: An Annotated Bibliography." Institute of Noetic Sciences, 1993. https://noetic.org/publication/spontaneous-remission-annotated-bibliography/.

Schrödinger, Erwin. *What Is Life? With Mind and Matter and Autobiographical Sketches*. London: Cambridge University Press, 1969.

Schwartz, Robert. *Your Soul's Plan*. Berkeley, CA: North Atlantic Books, 2009.

Science Learning Hub. "Preparing samples for the electron microscope." Science Learning Hub website, n.d. https://www.sciencelearn.org.nz/resources/500-preparing-samples-for-the-electron-microscope.

Seneff, Stephanie. *Toxic Legacy: How the Weedkiller Glyphosate Is Destroying Our Health and the Environment*. White River Junction, VT: Chelsea Green Publishing, 2021.

Shared Crossing Research Initiative. "Shared Death Experiences: A Little-Known Type of End-of-Life Phenomena Reported by Caregivers and Loved Ones." *American Journal of Hospice and Palliative Medicine*, Volume 38, Issue 12, 1479–87 (2021).

Sharma, Poonam, and Jim Tucker, MD. "Cases of the Reincarnation Type with Memories from the Intermission Between Lives." *Journal of Near-Death Studies*, 23 (2) (2004), 101, 118.

Sheldrake, Rupert. "Morphic Resonance: Research and Papers." Rupert Sheldrake website. https://www.sheldrake.org/research/morphic-resonance.

Shenton, Joan. *Positively False: Exposing the Myths Around HIV and AIDS*. London: Immunity Resource Foundation, 2015.

Siri, Aaron. "Proof Regarding the Clinical Trials Relied Upon by the FDA to License the Childhood Vaccines on the CDC Childhood Vaccine Schedule" within "What the 'Casual Cruelty' of Dr. Paul Offit Reveals." *Injecting Freedom*, August 3, 2023. https://aaronsiri.substack.com/p/what-the-casual-cruelty-of-dr-paul.

Sowell, Thomas. *Economic Facts and Fallacies*. New York: Basic Books, 2011.

Spivack, Barry, and Patricia Anne Saunders. *An Antidote to Violence*. Winchester, UK: Changemakers Books, 2020.

Stannard, David. *American Holocaust: Conquest of the New World*. Oxford: Oxford University Press, 1993.

Stevenson, Ian. *Children Who Remember Previous Lives: A Question of Reincarnation*. Jefferson, NC: McFarland, 2001.

Stevenson, Ian. *Where Reincarnation and Biology Intersect*. Westport, CT: Praeger, 1997.

Sunfellow, David. "Near-Death Experiences & Miraculous Healings." David Sunfellow's Substack website, April 16, 2023. https://sunfellow.substack.com/p/near-death-experiences-and-miraculous.

Swanson, Claude, PhD. *Life Force, the Scientific Basis: Breakthrough Physics of Energy Medicine, Healing, Chi and Quantum Consciousness*. Tucson, AZ: Poseidia Press, 2016.

TheWayFwrd. "OUR RESPONSE TO JJ COUEY." Bitchute video, January 19, 2023. https://www.bitchute.com/video/1ZJAZEkra4uI/.

Thorley, Bruce, and Jason Roberts. "Isolation and Characterization of Poliovirus in Cell Culture Systems." Springer Link website, n.d. https://link.springer.com/protocol/10.1007/978-1-4939-3292-4_4.

TLM4Columbia. "Voices in Virtue Lectures: Fr. Chad Ripperger — Demonology Function & Psychology." YouTube video, March 11, 2023. https://www.youtube.com/watch?v=A4Aq7WGIhzA.

The Tom Woods Show. "Ep. 2282 Do Viruses Exist?" The Tom Woods Show website, February 14, 2023. https://tomwoods.com/ep-2282-do-viruses-exist/#disqus_thread.

TrainofThoughts. "Maajid Nawaz – Mark Bailey – Why The Covid Virus Has Never Been Isolated – Jan 08 2023." Rumble video, January 8, 2023. https://rumble.com/v25m25v-maajid-nawaz-mark-bailey-why-the-covid-virus-has-never-been-isolated-jan-08.html.

Tran, Tony Ho. "The White House Admits It: We Might Need to Block the Sun to Stop Climate Change." *Daily Beast*, November 18, 2022. https://news.yahoo.com/white-house-admits-might-block-094049223.html.

Trebing, William. *Good-Bye Germ Theory: Ending a Century of Medical Fraud and How to Protect Your Family*. Dr. William P. Trebing, 2006.

Tressoldi, P. E. "Extraordinary Claims Require Extraordinary Evidence: The Case of Non-Local Perception, a Classical and Bayesian Review of Evidences." *Frontiers in Psychology* 2, no. 117 (2011).

Tulp, Sophia. "Experts say toxic pesticide DDT not linked to polio." AP, January 25, 2023. https://apnews.com/article/fact-check-polio-vaccine-ddt-pesticide-480376540979.

UK Health Security Agency. "FOI Response 25 March 2022." Fluoride Free Peel website, March 25, 2022. https://www.fluoridefreepeel.ca/wp-content/uploads/2022/05/UK-HSA-isolation-sequencing-methods-PACKAGE-redacted.pdf.

Utts, Jessica. "An Assessment of the Evidence for Psychic Functioning." *Journal of Parapsychology* 59, no. 4 (1995): 289–320.

van Lommel, Pim, and Bruce Greyson. "Critique of Recent Report of Electrical Activity in the Dying Human Brain." Invited commentary (preprint publication), 2023. https://iands.org/images/stories/pdf_downloads/vanLommel-Greyson-2023-Critique-Recent-Report-Electrical-Activity-Dying-Human-Brain.pdf.

Viroliegy. "Exposing the lies of Germ Theory and Virology Using Their Own Sources." Viroliegy website, n.d. https://viroliegy.com/2022/08/03/blindsided-by-rabies-with-michael-wallach-on-the-skeptico-podcast/.

von Magnus, P. and V. Bech. "A Pox-like Disease in Cynomolgus Monkeys." *Acta Pathologica Microbiologica Scandinavica*, 46, no. 2 (1959): 156–76.

Wahbeh, Helané. *The Science of Channeling: Why You Should Trust Your Intuition & Embrace the Force That Connects Us All.* Oakland, CA: New Harbinger Publications, 2021.

Wahbeh, H., L. Carpenter, and D. Radin. "A mixed methods phenomenological and exploratory study of channeling." *Journal of the Society for Psychical Research* 82, no. 3 (2018): 129–48.

Wallis, Paul. *Echoes of Eden: What Secrets of Human Potential Were Buried with Our Ancestors' Memories of ET Contact?* Paul Wallis Books, 2022.

Wallis, Paul. *The Eden Conspiracy: Ancient Memories of E.T. Contact and the Bible before God.* Paul Wallis Books, 2023.

Wallis, Paul. *Escaping from Eden: Does Genesis Teach That the Human Race Was Created by God or Engineered by ETs?* Axis Mundi Books, 2020.

Wallis, Paul. *The Scars of Eden: Has Humanity Confused the Idea of God with Memories of ET Contact?* Hampshire, UK: John Hunt Publishing, 2021.

War Room/DailyClout. "Pfizer Document Analysis Volunteers' Reports." War Room/DailyClout, 2022.

Waterson, A. P., and Lise Wilkinson. *An Introduction to the History of Virology.* Cambridge: Cambridge University Press, 1978.

West, Jim. *DDT/Polio: Virology vs. Toxicology.* Jim West, 2014.

West, Jim. "Pesticides and Polio: A Critique of Scientific Literature." harvoa.org website, August 14, 2015. https://harvoa.org/polio/overview.htm#_edn4.

West, Jim. "Pesticides and Polio: A Critique of Scientific Literature." Weston A. Price Foundation website, February 8, 2003. https://www.westonaprice.org/health-topics/environmental-toxins/pesticides-and-polio-a-critique-of-scientific-literature/#gsc.tab=0.

White, Michael. "Why Is the FDA Funded in Part by the Companies It Regulates?" University of Connecticut website, May 21, 2021. https://today.uconn.edu/2021/05/why-is-the-fda-funded-in-part-by-the-companies-it-regulates-2/#.

Wicker, Alden. *To Dye For: How Toxic Fashion Is Making Us Sick—and How We Can Fight Back.* New York: Putnam, 2023.

Wikipedia. "Tobacco mosaic virus." *Wikipedia*, accessed September 20, 2023. https://en.wikipedia.org/wiki/Tobacco_mosaic_virus. Accessed on September 20, 2023.

Williams, B. J. "Revisiting the Ganzfeld ESP Debate: A Basic Review and Assessment." *Journal of Scientific Exploration* 25, no. 4 (2011): 639–61.

Williams, Ulric, with Samantha Bailey. *Terrain Therapy*. Samantha Bailey, 2022.

Willow, Katherine. *German New Medicine: Experiences in Practice*. Katherine Willow, 2019.

Windbridge Research Center. "Completed Studies." Windbridge.org, n.d. https://www.windbridge.org/research/completed-studies/.

WISN. "'Dying of' vs. 'dying with': Medical Examiner explains COVID-19 difference." ABC WISN website, December 8, 2020. https://www.wisn.com/article/covid-19-dying-of-vs-dying-with-medical-examiner-explains-difference/34909031.

Wissenschafft Plus. N.d. https://wissenschafftplus.de/cms/de/empfehlungen.

World Health Organization. "Current U.S. Bird Flu Situation in Humans." CDC website, n.d. https://www.cdc.gov/flu/avianflu/inhumans.htm.

World Health Organization. "HIV and AIDS." World Health Organization website, July 13, 2023. https://www.who.int/news-room/fact-sheets/detail/hiv-aids.

World Health Organization. "Immunization Agenda 2030: A Global Strategy to Leave No One Behind." World Health Organization website, April 1, 2020. https://www.who.int/teams/immunization-vaccines-and-biologicals/strategies/ia2030.

World Health Organization. "Plague." WHO website, July 7, 2022. https://www.who.int/news-room/fact-sheets/detail/plague.

World Health Organization. "Severe Acute Respiratory Syndrome (SARS)." World Health Organization website, n.d. https://www.who.int/health-topics/severe-acute-respiratory-syndrome#tab=tab_1.

World Health Organization. "Tuberculosis." WHO website, April 21, 2023. https://www.who.int/news-room/fact-sheets/detail/tuberculosis.

Zakrzewski, Cat, and Joseph Menn. "5th Circuit finds Biden White House, CDC likely violated First Amendment." *Washington Post*, September 9, 2023. https://www.washingtonpost.com/technology/2023/09/08/5th-circuit-ruling-covid-content-moderation/.

Zane, Zachary. "How the Real-Life Rock Hudson From Hollywood Changed the AIDS Movement." *Men'sHealth*, May 1, 2020. https://www.menshealth.com/entertainment/a32228064/rock-hudson-aids/.

Zeck, Alec. "DEBUNKING THE NONSENSE." The Way Forward Unite Live website, July 21, 2022. https://unite.live/the-way-forward/the-way-forward?recording_id=1110.

INDEX

*Page numbers in *Italics* indicate illustrations.

E

N

U

V

ABOUT THE AUTHOR

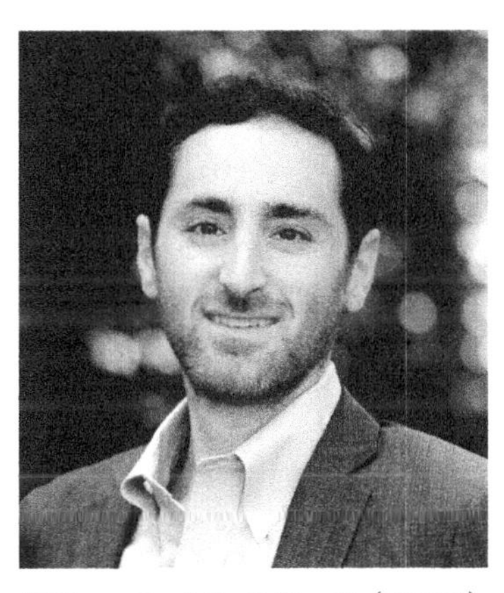

Mark Gober is the author of *An End to Upside Down Thinking* (2018), which won the Independent Publisher (IPPY) award for best science book of the year. He is also the author of *An End to Upside Down Living* (2020), *An End to Upside Down Liberty (2021), An End to Upside Down Contact* (2022), and *An End to the Upside Down Reset* (2023); and is the host of the podcast *Where Is My Mind?* (2019). Additionally, he serves on the board of the Institute of Noetic Sciences and the School of Wholeness and Enlightenment. Previously, Gober was a partner at Sherpa Technology Group in Silicon Valley and worked as an investment banking analyst in New York. He has been named one of *IAM's Strategy 300: The World's Leading Intellectual Property Strategists.*

Gober graduated magna cum laude from Princeton University, where he wrote an award-winning thesis on Daniel Kahneman's Nobel Prize–winning "Prospect Theory" and was elected a captain of Princeton's Division I tennis team.

Made in the USA
Coppell, TX
27 February 2026